STITCH YOUR OWN SILVER LININGS

SA

Please return or renew this item before the latest date shown below

Renewals can be made

by internet   www.fifedirect.org.uk/libraries

in person   at any library in Fife

by phone   08451 55 00 66

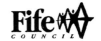

Fife
COUNCIL

Thank you for using your library

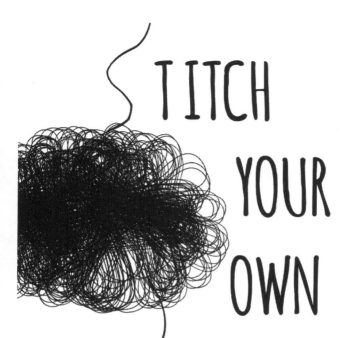

STITCH YOUR OWN SILVER LININGS

A BREAKTHROUGH GUIDE
TO HELPING YOURSELF
TO HAPPINESS –
NO MATTER WHAT

CHRISTINE L. CONROY

FOREWORD BY DR RYAN NIEMIEC

Matador
9 Priory Business Park
Kibworth Beauchamp
Leicestershire LE8 0RX, UK
Tel: (+44) 116 279 2299
Fax: (+44) 116 279 2277
Email: books@troubador.co.uk
Web: www.troubador.co.uk/matador

ISBN 978 1783063 345

British Library Cataloguing in Publication Data.
A catalogue record for this book is available from the British Library.

Printed and bound in the UK by TJ International, Padstow, Cornwall
Typeset in 11pt Aldine401 BT Roman by Troubador Publishing Ltd, Leicester, UK

To my heroes:
    Betty, Pat and Charlotte
        Such inspiration

To my saviours:
    Robin, Mitch and Josh
        Such gentlemen

    Love always

REMEMBER TO DOWNLOAD YOUR EXCLUSIVE GIFTS

FREE *'HELP YOURSELF TO HAPPINESS'* TRANSFORMATIONAL WORKBOOK HERE

www.ChristineLConroy/workbook

AND YOUR

FREE *'FIRST STEPS TO MEDITATION'* AUDIO HERE

www.ChristineLConroy/meditation

CONTENTS

Foreword

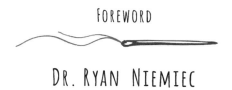

Dr. Ryan Niemiec

> It's not every day you get the opportunity to read empowering, authentic stories that blend with the latest science. Here's your chance.

One of the largest projects in the field of positive psychology was the creation of a universal classification of character strengths and virtues. This is known as the VIA Classification. It was accompanied by the VIA Survey, which is a user-friendly, scientific tool that measures these strengths of character. This was groundbreaking work that occurred shortly after the beginning of this millennium. Never before had there been a classification, based in science, that maps out a 'language' for understanding what is best in human beings – basic, positive psychological ingredients.

In one decade, this VIA work has found its way into the hands of millions of people reaching every country across the globe. Hundreds of scientists are now running research studies on character strengths. Thousands of coaches, counselors, business managers, and teachers are including the VIA Survey and practices designed to build character strengths in their work with clients, employees, and students. And, countless people in the general public are directly tapping into their signature character strengths to create their best life, reach their goals, develop greater happiness, and overcome life challenges.

This book, beautifully written by Christine L. Conroy, is another positive outgrowth of this work. Christine will not only take you on a journey through many of the elements of positive psychology but will pass along a number of practical tools. From appreciation letters to success journals to applying your strengths at work and at play, you will be able to concoct the exact recipe you need to cultivate happiness.

Most poignant are the stories. You will be brought to (inspired) tears by the story of Charlotte, be left in awe at the bravery of Pat, and learn nuggets of wisdom from Mum. Christine weaves these stories throughout the book like an expert seamstress. And, when I say you will 'feel' these positive emotions when reading this book, trust me. I mean it.

Not every sentence in this book should be viewed as a research-based finding. And it shouldn't be. Instead, Christine weaves astute observations and personal/professional experiences along with science-based tidbits. In one story, Christine shares how the use of two of her signature strengths (curiosity and humor) helped her to sustain her happy marriage. There's a lot to say about the importance of using your signature strengths (your highest qualities most core to who you are) at work, in school, and in your life in general, but applying them in marriage is a new area of research. Nevertheless, I fully agree with Christine. Learning to express who you are and what is best about you will help you embrace, connect, appreciate, and even cherish those you love the most. No doubt, science will eventually catch up with this wisdom and perhaps eventually find that a key factor in a flourishing marriage involves expressing your true self freely with your partner, and at the same time, savouring and appreciating who they are as well.

Character strengths are indeed a core part of this journey that Christine will take you on. You can spot them in every story and every page of this book. Test it yourself:

a) Choose any page (or story) at random;
b) Have the list of twenty-four VIA character strengths in hand (see page 118);
c) Read the page (or story);

d)   Spot the character strengths Christine is speaking to, directly or indirectly.

This is not only because of Christine's knowledge of the subject area and her talent for writing an engaging book, but also because our core character strengths are a natural fabric within our stories. They are at the essence of life. They are the steering wheel and the motor.

Through life experience, we can nourish and champion these best qualities within us. We can also stifle them. Christine shares how she needed to build up some aspects of her positivity and strength at times, and at other times, she full-out blasted her strengths and energy out there looking adversity in the eye, embracing beauty, climbing mountains of pain, and striving forward.

Sometimes people say that life is a collection of moments. We can also view life as a collection of stories. Perhaps one of our tasks in life is to understand and then embrace and express our stories? You have, at your fingertips, a collection of many of Christine's stories. Through her honest and forthright sharing, we learn just how precious, powerful, and transformative 'story' can be. Because Christine's sharing of herself and her family is so intimate and genuine, perhaps this will draw you to express your own story? We all have stories that matter.

In addition to being direct and honest about the good, the bad, the ugly, and the beautiful in her life, Christine's words flow from a place of love and hope. Warmth, genuineness, and optimism are present within the tragedies, the comedies, and everything in between. This is a recipe for inspiration. A recipe for meaningfulness. A recipe for how to stitch a silver lining.

Dr. Ryan Niemiec, Psy.D.
Education Director, VIA Institute on Character
Author: *Mindfulness and Character Strengths: A Practical Guide to Flourishing*
        Positive Psychology at the Movies: Using Films to Build Character
        Strengths and Well Being
November 2013

WE CAN ALL INCREASE OUR HAPPINESS LEVELS

'The UK and many other developed societies have experienced the paradox of getting richer, but not happier. For decades we have measured and analysed GDP (Gross Domestic Product) but have only recently recognized the merit in tracking our nation's happiness and life satisfaction.

We need to change our thinking about where true happiness comes from. Christine L. Conroy in *Stitch Your Own Silver Linings* gives us the tools to do just that. In this book Christine demonstrates that by thinking again about what we value in society we can all increase our happiness levels.

Christine's message that becoming 'happy first' equips us with the strength we need in order to cope with life's inevitable setbacks, comes from someone with powerful perspective given the challenges in her own life'.

Jo Swinson, MP
Founder of the All Party Parliamentary Group on Wellbeing Economics. Minister for Employment Relations and Consumer Affairs in the Department for Business, Innovation and Skills
December 2013

Introduction

Are you happy? Are you living the best life you could possibly live? Or, are you drifting through life hoping that tomorrow will be the day. Your time will come and that 'something' you are waiting for will happen and change your life completely. Do you think, 'If I could only do (you fill in the blank), I would be happy?' Or, 'If I could only have (you fill in the blank), I would be happy?' Perhaps you struggle along in a job you don't like, waiting for retirement when, finally, some happiness might be found before the long sleep? Alternatively, you might be experiencing personal problems or even dealing with tragedy right now that is making you think you will *never* be happy again.

If you have ever had any of these thoughts, you are not alone. However, I am here to tell you that your way of thinking is completely the wrong way round. Instead of thinking, 'If I could do this, I could have that and then I would be happy,' you need to think, 'If I could *be* happy, I could do this and then I could have that.' You need to be happy first.

Happiness will bring you the success you are looking for. You may well have heard that said before. The question is, how do you 'be happy first'? I am going to show you how. Even if, at the moment, you think you will never be happy again, stick with me. I will show you that no matter what your situation, you can be happy.

You do not have to wait to have, be, or do anything and you certainly don't have to wait for retirement, or any other time, to be

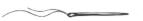

happy. You can help yourself to happiness right now. That's what this book is about. It is not filled with pleasing and wise but abstract quotations. Instead, it offers tried and tested practical actions that you can take today to take control of your own happiness.

ENJOY LIFE

My mission is to help you to be happy. I want you to be your own version of success. Most importantly, I want to help you to weather life's inevitable storms, and live life as it should be lived – enjoyed and not endured.

There was a time when I thought I would never be happy again. Cancer made me feel that way. Cancer threatened to destroy my life by tearing my loved ones away from me.

In the first chapter of this book, *Living the Life of Conroy – My Story*, I tell you a little about that. I want you to understand that I am not speaking to you about happiness from a place of charmed existence. I am neither wealthy nor beautiful. At least, not in the conventional sense. I do feel privileged. I have a strong, loving marriage and grown up children, who happen to be delightful people and the lights of my life. Other than that, I am an ordinary person thrown into extraordinary circumstances. Those circumstances taught me the purpose and meaning of my life and how to be happy, from the inside out. That's what I want to share with you.

CONROY WOMEN

I have the great pleasure of introducing you to three women who are my heroes, and without whom, there would be no Conroy. I call them my Conroy Women and I weave their stories through the book. I do this partly because I want you to get to know them (they are strong, funny and inspirational), but also to demonstrate that many of the ideas presented here were born from, or helped with, some harrowing, real life experiences.

There are many books out there on happiness or personal development and I have probably read most of them. When I read such books I find myself asking, 'But how does that relate to me and my life?' I have been conscious of that question, on your behalf, throughout the book. My story involves living and dying with cancer. Your story might not involve illness at all. Something else could be causing you to be in a bad place right now. Even if you are simply looking for more to life than you have already, this book will help you find it.

WHY ME

In addition to being a personal development coach, I am a university lecturer. The academic part of me struggles to accept anything I read unless there is strong evidence to support it. Equally, I don't expect you to accept what I suggest, purely on the basis of my experience alone. Thanks to exciting new sciences such as neuroscience (the study of the brain and nervous system), and positive psychology, we now know more than ever before about what makes us happy and what doesn't. These relatively new sciences provide us with the physical evidence to support what many coaches, spiritual leaders and, in some cases, even old wives, have been teaching for hundreds of years.

A brief introduction to positive psychology is included in Chapter Two. Through rigorous scientific investigation and experiment, positive psychology explores what we human beings need in order to perform at our best.

Traditional psychology focuses on human illness and disease. A psychologist takes a person from clinical illness, which would be minus five, to zero, where zero is normal (for want of a better word).

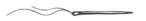

Positive psychology focuses on what makes us flourish as human beings, taking us from normal at zero, to plus five or more, which is flourishing. Most people are satisfied to coast through their lives feeling just 'okay' at 'zero'. That does not have to be you. It certainly isn't me. In fact, in honour of my heroes whose stories you will hear, I feel that I have a responsibility not to allow that to happen. I want to flourish and, yes, be happy.

UNDERSTANDING HAPPINESS

Most people have a hopelessly vague notion about what happiness is. They say they want to be happy but don't really know what that is. It's a little bit like saying to a taxi driver, 'I want to go somewhere but I don't know where.' When I talk about the science of positive psychology, I give a succinct definition of happiness that gives us something more tangible to work with. We take a surprising look at what makes us happy and what has been shown not to. Here too, I will offer scientific evidence demonstrating that you are in control of your own happiness and wellbeing.

It is liberating. You do not need to rely on anything or anybody to make you happy. Therefore, no-one and nothing has the power to take it away from you. Please do not assume that I am all about 'Pollyanna, always positive' cheeriness. I am not. I tackle negative emotions head on and we deal with them throughout the book. Finally, in this science chapter, I explain precisely why it is important that you make the effort to be happy and how it will give you the edge in every area of your life.

THE CONROY CONCEPT

Once you know a little about the Who – me and my Conroy Women

– and the What and the Why of happiness, you will discover the How in Chapters Three and Four. These two chapters cover the introduction to the Conroy Concept of Happiness and Well-being. The Concept gives you a solid foundation from which to build a strong, long-lasting happiness level that will enable you to live the best life you could possibly live.

For ease of expression and understanding, this part of the guide is organized around the word CONCEPT. I offer tried and tested suggestions in seven key areas about how to raise your happiness levels. Personal stories demonstrate the practical applications of these ideas and I include exercises to help you put them to use in your own life. Some of these exercises will give immediate benefits, some will take practice. I say to you as I do to my clients, choose the exercises that appeal to you the most. If you feel uncomfortable with any of them, ignore them. I would ask, however, that you don't make the mistake of ignoring the more simple exercises. Sometimes the simple ones are the most effective. The Conroy Concept itself is simple but not always easy. You have to be willing to invest time and effort in yourself, but you can make it fun. I promise it will pay dividends.

Underpinning the Conroy Concept are two things that I believe are essential to your lasting happiness: Forgiveness and Appreciation. I discuss these in Chapter Five.

FORGIVENESS AND APPRECIATION

Has anyone ever done something so mean or bad to you that you still feel angry every time you think about it? Are there people you know who are no longer part of your life because they did something in the past to hurt you? If there are, you need to know it's probably making you ill. You might want to forgive these people but don't know how. Forgiveness is another much written about subject, but nobody actually explains how to do it. Although it is the most personal and possibly the most difficult thing to do, forgiveness is also the most rewarding once it is accomplished. By the end of Chapter Five, you will be more open and willing to forgive, which will make the whole process easier for you.

Appreciation is much easier than forgiveness. Unfortunately, all too often we seem to forget about it. The nature of our fast-paced world, the uncertain economic situation, and any number of other things, means we spend most of our time worrying about what is wrong in our lives. We barely notice the things that are right. If, at present, your response to that is 'nothing *ever* goes right for me', this section of the book will show you how to change your focus. As you start to pay attention to the things that go well in your life, you will be surprised at how quickly they start to multiply.

Once you have reached that point in the book, you will know how to help yourself to happiness and will already be seeing some changes in your life. The thing is, I don't want you to see *some* changes in your life, I want you to see your life transformed. I want you to make the changes that will result in permanent, higher levels of happiness that will give you a much deeper, richer experience of life.

In order to do that, we take a slight detour in the second part of the book, and here you will need to be ruthlessly honest with yourself. Over the years, you may have acquired some negative beliefs about yourself and your capabilities. Often, these beliefs lurk deep inside you, ready to rise to the surface just in time to sabotage your success. Sometimes they are there constantly, seemingly laughing at you. These feelings need to be routed out and addressed. I am talking about low self-esteem and lack of confidence, possibly with some shyness thrown in. While I don't pretend to be able to rid you of feelings of low self-esteem in two chapters of a book, I do hope to bring it fully to your conscious attention.

I look at some of the latest thinking on self-esteem and include

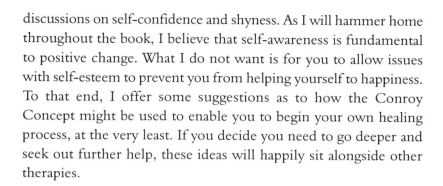

discussions on self-confidence and shyness. As I will hammer home throughout the book, I believe that self-awareness is fundamental to positive change. What I do not want is for you to allow issues with self-esteem to prevent you from helping yourself to happiness. To that end, I offer some suggestions as to how the Conroy Concept might be used to enable you to begin your own healing process, at the very least. If you decide you need to go deeper and seek out further help, these ideas will happily sit alongside other therapies.

SUCCESS

In the final chapters of the book, instead of looking at things that are holding you back, we discuss things that will help to catapult you to greater levels of happiness and success. We will unearth resources in you that you never knew you had. What's more, we look at ways to develop and harness those resources to make your life the best possible life for you.

With raised happiness levels, we also tackle head on what to do when things go wrong. There is no denying that bad things happen to even the happiest of people. Things will go wrong – storm clouds will gather. Problems are a part of life, so let's look at what to do about them. Through reading *Stitch Your Own Silver Linings,* you will learn to change your thinking. You will gain a greater understanding of positive emotions and how to train yourself to be and feel positive. Genuine positive thinking will then become second nature. And finally, we collect together all the tools you need to stitch your own silver lining on every cloud.

Being happy needs to be nurtured. It requires your constant, loving attention. I stress throughout the book that it is your thoughts and your actions that determine how happy you are. You need to 'practise happy' until you get the Happiness Habit. I will give you

some ideas to help you, at long last, move forward into your new happy and fulfilled way of living.

The Dalai Lama says, 'Happiness is not something ready made. It comes from your own actions.'

As you will see, you really are in control of your own happiness and well-being.

CHAPTER ONE

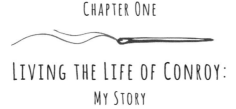

LIVING THE LIFE OF CONROY:
MY STORY

'Sorry I didn't come to yesterday's class. I couldn't get outa bed coz I was depressed.' That was the reason given to me by an undergraduate student for his absence from one of my lectures. He was neither lying nor joking. Although not part of the curriculum, following similar disturbing conversations with a number of the students, I decided that a discussion on well-being was needed. It seemed that many of my students were unhappy. At the age of eighteen, some were dissatisfied with their lot, others disillusioned with life, while some were actually clinically depressed. I was shocked. I raised the issue as part of my Competitive Edge Programme, designed to help students prepare to compete in an increasingly difficult employment market. I didn't talk about happiness because that term is often considered slightly frivolous and not always taken seriously. Instead, I talked about subjective well-being. It sounds far more academic and much more appropriate for an intellectual setting. As it happens, I like the term subjective well-being. It describes well what I mean by happiness.

One day during the Competitive Edge seminar, a student commented, 'Well, it's okay for you to talk about happiness and well-being. You have everything you want: married with a family, a good career, a flash car. It's easy to feel good when everything is going well.'

He stopped me in my tracks because I thought he had a point. This student didn't know me or my story. I had been his lecturer for a few weeks, that's all. Why should I be talking to him about life in this way? With that in mind, I am going to, briefly, tell you my story here. I want you to understand who I am and why I am passionate about helping you to increase your happiness and well-being and enjoy your life more.

The Early Years

I was a mistake; born in an industrial town in the north of England to parents who could ill afford a fourth child. Yet, there I was. I spent eight wonderful years as the baby of the family. Two older brothers and an older sister spoilt me and, naturally, I loved every minute of it. Until… another mistake in the form of a baby sister arrived. I developed a mysterious tummy bug. It lasted for weeks and hurt particularly badly whenever 'the baby' had adoring visitors. I soon realized this usurper was here to stay. It took a while longer to understand that I had better just get used to it.

My parents married far too young in life and their marriage ended almost as soon as it began. Nevertheless, they stayed together for twenty-two turbulent years before they divorced. Twelve months after that, as I turned thirteen, my father was killed in an accident. I remember little about him except that his bullying made our lives thoroughly miserable. Following the divorce, my mother, desperate never to see his face again, destroyed all photographs of him so I have even lost the memory of what my father looked like. On the other hand, I distinctly remember his smell. For most of my childhood he drove huge articulated wagons for a living. Working hard and long hours, his nightly journey home from work included a visit to the local bar. Consequently, he always carried with him a smell of diesel and alcohol that I actually found quite pleasant. One whiff of either smell and even now, some fifty years later, I am catapulted back to childhood.

Terrible Teenager

Left to raise her family alone, my mother ruled with an iron fist. At least, she ruled *me* with an iron fist. I felt trapped, frustrated and angry. I had a rebellious streak in me which, in retrospect, I thank God stayed with me. It has served me well.

At twenty-one years old, I had successfully completed a secretarial course at a local college. Since leaving school at fifteen, I hadn't been satisfied with the jobs I'd had and now looked for more fulfilling work. I was still living at home and every morning Mum would turn me out of the house warning, 'Don't come home until you have a job.' Unfortunately, day after day I did return without work and it caused major friction between us. One day, and I can't even remember where it came from, I read a book that changed my life. *The Power of Positive Thinking,* by Norman Vincent Peale.

At that time, in an effort to understand my upbringing and its effects on me, I could always be found with a heavyweight psychology book in my bag. At one company where I worked, this became a standing joke. While the other girls read *Women's Weekly* or *Cosmopolitan* magazines, I read books with titles such as *Games People Play* and *I'm OK, You're OK.* I wanted answers and these books went some way towards addressing that need. *The Power of Positive Thinking,* though, was unlike anything I had read.

As a child, I had always believed in the power of magic and here, I thought, was the proof. The solution to my problems. I simply had to decide what I wanted, visualize it, have faith and… *voilá,* magic would happen. And happen it did. For a few nights before going to sleep, I imagined myself in an office typing. I imagined it with such clarity that I could almost feel my fingers stroking the keys. I imagined coming home to Mum and, finally telling her: 'Hey, I've got a job!'

I went to sleep with thoughts of success on my mind and woke up with renewed enthusiasm. A few days later Mum gave me a newspaper. I saw that she had drawn a huge red circle around an advertisement for a secretarial position. It was at a local company. In an instant, I knew this was what I had been waiting for. I made the call immediately and within a week I had started my new job.

The chain of events was so amazing that it was almost spooky. It was definitely spooky when, eighteen months later, I married the man who had interviewed me for that job. It became magic when, some twelve years later, we bought the company together. But I am ahead of myself now.

Raising five children alone must have been demanding for Mum, but she was always strong. Whenever she saw us struggling with something she would say, 'Where there's a will, there's a way.' Or, 'You can do anything you set your mind to.' I went on to live my life with those words in mind.

Throughout my teenage years the relationship with my family was fraught. During that time I left home more than once, but was twenty-one before I left for the final time. My relationship with Mum had deteriorated so badly that I wouldn't see her again for eight years. That time apart changed us both. I matured and she softened. We met again after I had my first child and slowly began to rebuild our relationship. From this time, my relationship with my little sister, Pat, also blossomed.

With eight years between us, Pat and I had never been close growing up. When I left home, she was only thirteen years old. Now, she was a young woman of twenty-one. It was only now that we started to get to know each other. One night we were talking and she told me a story that painted in colourful detail what life was like for her at that time. She said:

'I was undercover in one of the local nightclubs and had a gun pulled on me by a gang member. I knew if I created a fuss he would panic and maybe fire the gun into the crowded club. I let him think he'd frightened me and that he'd got away with it. I walked away. When I got to the foyer of the club I arranged a single file walk out of all the patrons of the club. (This is where the people are allowed out only one at a time.) When the 'perp' got to the door he was faced with an armed response unit… pointing guns straight at him. He was arrested and charged with possession of the gun and the drugs and some other stuff.'

My 'baby' sister was a fearless undercover officer for the local vice squad.

By the time Pat reached her teenage years, my mother had mellowed dramatically, and anyway, she didn't challenge the house rules like I did. Instead she said, 'I was so much smarter than you. I knew how to "play the game" to get what I wanted.' Consequently, she and my mother enjoyed a much better relationship. Life was good for Pat at this time. She absolutely adored her job and was in a happy long-term relationship with a man who also worked for the police force.

I was discovering a new person. We were all different. Only now did we begin to enjoy each other.

At thirty-three, I was happily married to Robin, and we had brought three gorgeous children into the world. Two delightful boys and a beautiful little girl made our family complete.

My husband and I have blonde-ish hair but all three children had that lovely white-blonde hair that, unfortunately, often disappears as children grow. One time while on holiday, we were eating at a restaurant when the waitress approached our table. Smiling, she turned to her colleague and shouted, 'Hey look, here's that beautiful family from the beach I was telling you about this morning.' All the diners turned to look at us. Although I blushed from head to toe, I thought I might burst with pride. I didn't think I could be any happier.

Robin and I were hugely driven and goal-orientated. We ran a successful furniture design business together and employed more than sixty people. The nature of the business dictated that we work during the evenings and, for a long time, we opened the showroom seven days a week. Not so much a job as a way of life. When we married, everyone warned us against working together, telling us it was bad for a relationship. For a while, we listened. I went off to do other things but we missed working together. It wasn't long before I was back on board. We made a good team. We worked long and hard but we were building a great life and the rewards were good. Our home was lovely. We employed a nanny to help with the children. We drove expensive cars and enjoyed wonderful holidays. We were well on our way to achieving all the things that society values and sees as success.

Then, brick-by-agonising-brick, life began to fall apart.

The Twilight Zone

By the time I was thirty-seven, my mum, my sister Pat, and my seven-year old daughter Charlotte, had all been diagnosed with cancer.

The cancers were different and totally unrelated. I don't know what the chances of that happening are but there is certainly no rule book on how to deal with it. Cancer attacked my mum's lungs. My sister had Hodgkin's lymphoma, which is cancer of the lymph nodes, and my daughter, osteosarcoma or bone cancer. It came out of nowhere – a bit like being smacked in the face with a cricket bat.

We were hurled into, what we later christened, The Twilight Zone – life, but not as we knew it. We went through the motions of living but existed in a weird, altered state brought about by abject fear; never knowing from one minute to the next what was going to happen or to whom. One minute we might be out shopping for dinner or organising the kids for school and the next, bang! Gut wrenching, all consuming fear. We lived inside a house of cards afraid to breathe too deeply in case we blew it all down.

To Treat or not To Treat

My sister suffered dreadfully from the after-effects of the chemotherapy treatment of her lymphoma. At this stage, Pat and Mum lived together. So sick and ill on some days, Pat refused to let anyone see her in that state. Mum cared for her 24-hours a day. Mercifully, after going through hell and back, Pat lived to fight another day. What we didn't know then was that her chemotherapy treatment would make her infertile, weaken her heart and, later, go on to be a contributory factor to causing breast cancer.

An operation to remove part of Mum's lung gave her some respite. It wasn't long, though, before a persistent pain in her back signalled the cancer's return. She asked me to go to see her one day and told me that she had decided to refuse chemotherapy treatment. The distressing experience of nursing Pat through her treatment was part of this determined decision. Mum asked for my support, which I gave unequivocally. Then I went home and wept. She went through unnecessary soul searching to make that decision because, in the end, chemotherapy was not offered to her – the disease had spread too far.

Not Only one in a Million

Charlotte's condition was the most perplexing for the medical profession. Her condition was so rare that, to their knowledge, nobody had ever presented with her symptoms. She was one on her own. She had a bone tumour in her left arm. As if this was not enough, there was apparently a sinister, underlying and unknown condition that caused the cancer in the first place. That discovery took the 'treat-or not-to-treat using chemotherapy' decision for Charlotte out of our hands. It was not an option because it might kill her. There was a treatment open to us… but it was unthinkable.

In the end we had no choice. I wonder, how would *you* tell your beautiful, vivacious, charming, funny, sporty and active seven-year-old daughter that the doctor is going to cut off her arm?

How we laboured over that question. 'What if we say this? What if we do it this way? What if we have the whole family with us? How might she react? What will we do then? What if? What if? What if?' On and on. We discussed it at great length. The hospital offered us meetings with social workers, counsellors, and other therapists. All of whom were available to help us have this horrific conversation with our little girl.

We were acutely aware that before we spoke to Charlotte, Robin and I had to get our own acts together. Meaning that we had to explore our own emotions first and attempt to deal with them. We had to present a united front that would allow Charlotte to feel confident and, somehow, unafraid. She needed to feel secure, loved and assured that everything was going to be alright. To be able to do that for her, we had to believe it first. Or, at least, do an excellent job of appearing to believe it.

I understand this is a strange comparison but I remember as children, my brothers, sisters and I loved thunder and lightning. Whenever the sky darkened and the rain bounced off the ground, Mum would be with us expectantly looking out of the windows. Excited, we watched waiting to see the lightning and hear the thunder. It was thrilling. However, whilst we were thrilled by the weather, the mother in the house next door was in the cupboard underneath the stairs, terrified. And where do you think her children were? Right there with her, underneath the stairs screaming in fear.

This memory informed my parenting when I became a mother. When something happens to make a child feel uncertain, they look first to you for your reaction, and they follow your lead. If they see you frightened and upset, they become frightened and upset too.

ENOUGH IS ENOUGH

With this story in mind, Robin and I spent time thrashing out our own concerns. Remembering that the operation would save Charlotte's life helped us to be positive. One evening amidst all of this turmoil, I pottered about in the bathroom waiting for Charlotte to finish her bath. She was scooping up bubbles in her cupped hands and blowing them everywhere. I was miles away thinking about other things. I snapped to attention when she said, 'Mummy, my arm hurts me so much now that last night I was awake all the time. If I wake up tonight, can I come into your bed?'

Her painkillers were strong but, obviously, now not powerful enough. My heart split right down the middle. I decided enough was enough. Without giving it a second thought, I said, 'I wonder if it would be possible for the doctors to take your arm off? That way, the cancer we talked about couldn't spread anywhere else and you would not be in any pain.'

That opened up the conversation. No big deal, no meetings and no fuss. We chatted calmly about the possibility whilst getting her dry from the bath and putting on her pyjamas. Her concerns were twofold: would she still be able to swim and ride horses, and would she look silly with only one arm?

Oh yes. And how, exactly, would they take her arm off?

The swimming and horse riding were no problem. Would she look silly? I opened her pyjama jacket, tucked her left arm inside and stood her in front of the mirror. 'What do you think?' I asked. 'Does it look silly?'

We decided it didn't look silly. It looked like she had a broken arm. Later, we told Robin and the boys about our conversation. The

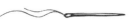

boys, who were almost six and eleven years old at the time, were, and remain, my saviours. They kept us sane. Both sensitive, both intelligent, and both protective and caring of their sister, always.

A FAMILY DAY OUT

Mitch, our eldest son, suggested that the next day we all go down to the shopping centre. Charlotte could tuck her arm in her coat as we had done with the pyjama jacket and we could watch to see if anyone looked at her. It was a risk but Charlotte loved the idea. The next day, off we went. When we arrived at the shops, Charlotte giggled with glee at the prospect of what she was about to do. I was nervous and ready to terminate the mission should anything hurtful happen.

My heart was in my mouth as Charlotte and I walked along. The boys followed watching the reactions of passers-by. Afterwards, we took seats in a cafe and chatted about the results.

People did look twice at her. Between us, we came to the conclusion that it was okay to do that because she did look a little different. We also decided that anyone who stared at her was downright rude and obviously didn't know how to behave. She could dismiss them. Off we went again. This time the boys sang out 'okay' when someone merely looked and 'rude' when they stared.

A strange way to spend the morning, I agree. But we made it fun, and it did work to put Charlotte's mind, somewhat, at ease.

The next time we used role play around the reactions of others came after her operation. Charlotte was due back at school. Our concern then was how the other children were going to react when they saw her. At the time her 'little' arm was still quite thickly wrapped in bandages, but she was healing well and keen to see her friends. As a family, once again, we came together to discuss the possibilities. We had to consider that somebody might say something that would upset or hurt her and we wanted to prepare her for that.

As light-hearted and gently as possible, we came up with all the name calling we could think of, from one arm bandit to the big nasty – freak. It sounds harsh now in the telling but we wanted her to own the language, to be familiar with it and understand the reasons someone might use it. If that's at all possible.

They say children can be cruel. Well, not these children. The school handled it marvellously and so did the children. They were only ever kind, thoughtful and helpful. It is sad to say but if Charlotte has ever suffered from the cruelty of others, it has been at the hands of the grown-ups, not the children.

HAMMER AND CHISEL

Back to addressing the final concern about how, exactly, the surgeon would take Charlotte's arm off. This proved to be more difficult. We didn't know the answer to that question so I suggested we ask the doctor when we went to see him. I let Charlotte ask the question.

Three different visits and three different doctors later we still didn't have the answer. Everyone spoke to her in that, child-patronizing way that always begins in a soft but high-pitched tone. 'Well, Charlotte…' followed by, 'And when you wake up, it will all be over.' One doctor almost broke down in tears as she spoke and I had to rescue her by suggesting, 'Don't worry, we'll speak to the surgeon.' So, that's what happened. We requested a meeting with the surgeon and he was excellent. In fairness, I had pre-warned him that Charlotte wanted the full story, in detail. That's precisely what we got. Robin and I held our breath as Charlotte was given a blow-by-blow account. The surgeon gave us a detailed description of the necessary equipment, using hacking and sawing terminology that she could understand. It was gruesome. Charlotte listened intently and then said, 'Will I be able to see my arm once you have taken it off?' I thought I might faint.

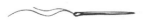

Without missing a heartbeat, the surgeon explained that the arm had to go away for analysis of the tumour. We let out long sighs of relief.

As he walked away, the surgeon silently mouthed to us, 'How did I do?'

Brilliantly. He did brilliantly and we were so thankful. 'Knowledge is power,' as the saying goes, and it goes for children too.

The Sword of Damocles

Charlotte's left arm was amputated just above the elbow. After the operation the tumour went off for analysis and that's when the phone calls started. We had been home from the hospital for about a week. The consultant rang telling us that Charlotte had a particular disease. I can't remember the name of it now but it doesn't matter. A few days later we received another call telling us they now thought she had something else. This went on for days. Each disease they came up with was ghastly and each one worse than the last. We lived in fear of the phone ringing. One morning Mitch came into the kitchen to find me weeping beside a ringing telephone simply unable to pick it up. We never did receive a firm diagnosis for Charlotte. We were told, however, that her life expectancy, even after the amputation, was twelve months, if we were lucky.

We lived under the sword of Damocles and it was hell. Each time Charlotte sneezed, coughed, refused to eat, or slept too long, we thought, this is it. The strain was too much to bear. We hit our lowest point.

Time for an Attitude Change

Twelve months later we were blessed that Charlotte was still with us, but by that time we had lost everything else: the family business, the nanny, the cars, and the holidays. Thankfully, our home was safe.

In his book *Man's Search for Meaning*, the Holocaust survivor Viktor Frankl says*:*

'Everything can be taken from a person but one thing: the last of human freedoms – to choose one's attitude in any given set of circumstances… to choose one's own way.'

Robin and I had both studied the human condition and personal development literature. I had spent a lifetime reading spiritual teachings and I had read *Man's Search for Meaning*. It was time we changed our attitude. We had three fantastic kids to take care of and we needed to get our lives back. Once we had finally reached that conclusion, we began to instinctively and purposefully live our lives putting into practice the things we had learned. Some of these ideas were the exact same ones that positive psychologists are now saying help to make us happier and lead to success. I would go further by adding they are ideas that help to build resilience. Tragedy, disaster, loss, or misery of some kind befalls us all at some times in our lives. We need to build resilience to be able to deal with that and come back even stronger than before.

My family is living proof that these ideas work. My mum and sister encouraged me to write them down and I gave them the umbrella term of the Conroy Concept. Gradually, step by step, Robin and I moved forward. We went on to have a different life; a life that allowed us to spend time with our kids and each other. Rather than aim for society's imposed ideas of what success is, we decided what success meant for us at that time, and aimed for that instead. That led us to a much richer and more fulfilling life than anything we had before.

Talking about this time so briefly seems almost to demean the experience and I certainly don't mean to. Contrary to what my students may have thought, I want you to understand that when I talk about happiness and well-being, it is because I have lived the

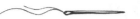

'life of Conroy' and not the 'life of Riley'. It is because I have discovered how to move through the toughest of times and still be happy. I have discovered how to allow that happiness to help me achieve my own versions of success and I want you to discover that too.

If you are dealing with heartbreak or challenges of any kind, the loss of a loved one, illness, finances, career challenges, or even persistent more mundane difficulties, I know from first-hand experience how that feels. I don't pretend to know exactly how *you* feel. I learned through coaching others that two people can experience exactly the same thing and feel completely differently about it. What I do know is that by following the Conroy Concept of Happiness and Well-being along with some of the other ideas in this book, you will breakthrough your challenges quicker and emerge stronger. You will be ready to move forward and help yourself to a happier and more fulfilling life, safe in the knowledge that when trouble comes calling again, it too shall pass.

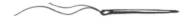

Chapter Two

The Science of Happiness:
Positive Psychology

Positive psychology is a relatively new science. It argues that human excellence and well-being are as relevant and important as mental disease and distress.

About fifteen years ago a number of psychologists believed there to be something missing from their discipline. Traditional psychology was excellent at focusing on human problems and how to put them right, but some psychologists felt a more balanced picture of human nature was needed. Improving the human condition is not only about eradicating problems but also about increasing well-being. This is now achieved by developing and applying tried and tested interventions or exercises and actions to increase the well-being of ordinary people. That is, those without clinical conditions.

In a nutshell, positive psychology is the science of happiness and well-being. The study of optimal functioning. Positive traits, such as character strengths, are considered along with creating positive institutions, such as schools and businesses.

Personal growth and well-being is my field and I have a special interest in positive psychology. Back at university, when I discovered that my students needed guidance with personal development, I knew I was the one to help them. I understood instinctively that happy students learn better. I also knew that if I were to persuade the university to allow me to give seminars in this area, I needed an official qualification. I undertook intensive training to become a personal development coach and, in addition, studied positive psychology. As part of my studies, in 2009 I attended the first World Congress on Positive Psychology in Philadelphia, USA. It was a revelation for me.

There in Philadelphia, immersed in the ideas of some of the world's most eminent psychologists (Martin Seligman, Philip Zimbardo and Ed Diener, amongst others), I was truly inspired. Previous studies and experience had certainly given me the tools to help people. Now, the research and experiments undertaken by these positive psychologists finally gave me the scientific evidence to support much of what I was already teaching. It was a turning point for me. I felt ready to become more involved in the personal transformational world.

Positive psychology is not an ideological movement or a quick fix for anything. It is an applied science offering interventions and assessments that are a valuable addition to my coaching toolbox and it underpins most of what I do.

WHAT IS HAPPINESS?

Before answering that question, let me ask you something. What makes you happy? Do you have an answer? Some people simply don't know. Sometimes when I ask that question I get responses such as dinner with friends, buying new clothes, or losing weight. Many people confuse happiness with pleasure.

Pleasure is important and we will talk about it, but pleasure is fleeting. When I talk about happiness, I mean something longer lasting. According to positive psychology, the definition of happiness or subjective well-being is:

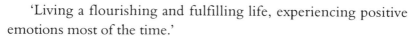

'Living a flourishing and fulfilling life, experiencing positive emotions most of the time.'

A person who lives a flourishing life, experiencing positive emotions *most* of the time is what is defined as a happy person. True happiness is not about positivity all the time. That would be unnatural.

Negative emotions are important to us. Anger, sadness and fear have an important part to play in our lives. There can be valid causes to feel worried, frightened or angry. These negative emotions alert us to danger or to the fact that something is wrong. To be able to sense problems on the horizon and prepare for them is prudent. Unfortunately, too many of us allow negativity to take over our thinking and, therefore, our lives.

When my family was wading through The Twilight Zone, negative emotions dominated our lives on a daily basis and for prolonged periods of time. This lead to a downward spiral resulting in a sense of hopelessness that, for a while, rendered us ineffective in our lives. Unchecked, negative emotions are unhealthy at best and dangerous at worst.

So, is it possible for us to become happier than we are? Can we become the happy person the positive psychologists are talking about? Well, thankfully, the answer to both of those questions is a resounding 'yes'. That's what this book is about, showing you how to do that.

You might be asking yourself: why bother? Why is it important? And why is happiness such a hot subject right now? Because, it certainly *is* a hot subject. In 1972 the King of Bhutan, Jigme Singye Wangchuk, had a sophisticated survey instrument developed to measure his population's level of well-being. The king coined the term 'gross national happiness' and everyone laughed at him. They are not laughing at him now. In April 2012 a meeting at the United Nations Headquarters in New York took place. More than 600 attendees from governments, business, spiritual, and academic groups came together to discuss Happiness. It was the first meeting

of its kind, putting well-being at the heart of economic progress. And here's why:

Numerous studies show that happy people are:

1) More successful in relationships and marriage

Happy people are more sociable and liked by others. They are more likely to be charitable and willing to see another's point of view. They have more friends and more social support and are more likely to get married and stay married.

2) More successful in business and finance

They are more productive at work, are more creative, and are better leaders and negotiators. And they earn more.

3) More successful in health

They cope better with stress and trauma; have stronger immune systems, are physically healthier and even live longer.

Imagine a country where families stay together without the need for state intervention, where businesses thrive, employment is high and caring capitalism is the order of the day. Imagine a country whose citizens are physically and mentally healthier, therefore greatly reducing the burden on the country's health care systems. No wonder governments are investigating.

The oldest person in Great Britain, at present, is 113 years old. On average we can all expect to live into our eighties. Fantastic news, but surely we want to live longer *and* be happy and healthy.

Before I talk about how to do that we need to look at what determines happiness levels. Positive psychologist Sonja Lyubomirsky calls it the 'forty per cent solution'. It is going to surprise you.

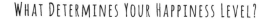

WHAT DETERMINES YOUR HAPPINESS LEVEL?

Imagine that your happiness level is represented by a lovely big chocolate cake. Fifty per cent of your happiness cake is determined by genetics. You inherit this from your parents and there is nothing you can do about it. Called the set point, it's the baseline level of happiness to which you will return even after major setbacks or great successes.

The next figure is possibly the most surprising and counter-intuitive. Only ten per cent of your happy cake is determined by circumstances. Yes, you read that right. Only ten per cent of your happiness level is determined by whether you are: healthy or unhealthy, beautiful or not, even rich or poor.

Consider this: In the Western world over the last fifty years our general living circumstances have improved beyond recognition.

At home, as a child, Monday was wash day. That's when mum did all the laundry and I had to help. I hated Mondays. Mum would wash the clothes and have to squeeze out the excess water before hanging them out to dry. Each item was laboriously fed through a clothes mangle or wringer. I had to stand at the other side of the mangle and catch the clothes coming through. It was difficult, tedious and dangerous. As a child, Robin almost lost his index finger tackling this job for his mum. His poor little finger went through the mangle and the tip of it is now quite flat.

Bath time was no easier. My brother, sister, and I would share the water in a huge tin bath placed in front of the fire. Mum trudged backwards and forwards to fill the bath with buckets of water from the kitchen sink. The youngest of the three, so the last one in the water, I had to suffer a lukewarm or often freezing cold bath. Another 'joy' to be endured was traipsing down the backyard to an outside toilet.

During the summer, my friends and I spent our days playing in the back streets with little more than sticks and stones to play with. I remember sitting for hours rolling tar balls from the melted tar on the road. We couldn't afford plasticine.

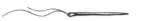

You probably have similar memories yourself or have heard such stories from your family. Life has certainly improved since those days.

Today, most of you reading this book will have washing machines and tumble driers that all but do the laundry for you. In your homes there will be untold labour saving gadgets that make your life easier and fantastic electronic gizmos for your entertainment. I don't know, but I imagine few of you have to traipse outside the house to go to the bathroom.

Income has risen along with our standard of living and since the 1950s our lives have become much easier. We are surely much happier now than we were back then. Not true.

In fact, ten times more people suffer from depression now than they did in 1945. Major depression is the number one psychological disorder in the Western world. What's worse is the fastest rate of increase in depression is found in young people. Predictions are that by 2020 it will follow only heart disease as *the* most disabling condition. Given that only ten per cent of depression has a biological cause, how can this be so?

Largely, it is because we are taught to look for happiness in the wrong places. When we can't find it, we become disillusioned and are led to believe there must be something wrong with us.

Society still values and views success almost exclusively in material terms. And yet, the facts speak for themselves. Once a certain amount of money is earned, increases in income do not make that much difference to happiness levels. Basic needs must be met, and a bit more for a few extras. After that, the happiness more money brings levels out.

How many times have you heard stories about lottery winners who say they are scarcely happier after the win than before? Or even worse, that it ruined their lives. Maybe that's because they didn't earn the money and so are unaccustomed to dealing with it? Possibly, but not necessarily.

In 2005 an American newspaper surveyed 792 wealthy businessmen, 500 of whom were worth over a million dollars. More than half of them said more wealth did not bring more happiness. A third of those worth more than ten million dollars said money brought more problems than it was worth. Another study carried out as far back as 1985 showed that the richest Americans reported only slightly higher happiness levels than their office staff.

I am not saying that all wealthy people are unhappy people or that money can't buy happiness. In fact, there is a saying: 'Anyone who says money can't buy happiness – is not spending it right!' Another pearl of wisdom from Mum: 'There are only two reasons to have lots of money: one is to travel, and the other is to help people.'

What I am saying is that you will not find happiness by chasing money purely for material gain. According to psychology, the explanation for that is adaptation.

ADAPTATION

We adapt to our circumstances. Having this conversation with my son, Josh, he told me, 'I am sorry Mum, but if I had a fabulous, bright red Ferrari parked on the drive right now it would make me incredibly happy.' Yes, it probably would, for a few weeks, perhaps even months. After that, he would begin to take his beautiful car for granted. The novelty of driving it around would wear off. Soon, he would need a bigger, better car to give him the same thrill.

Has this ever happened to you? I'm sure it has. I remember moving to our current home in the country. I thought it absolutely perfect and was delightfully happy. It wasn't long, however, before I wanted changes made to improve it. Of all of our life circumstances, material goods are what we take for granted the most and the quickest. This sets us off on an endless search for more and bigger

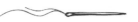

and better. Positive psychologists call this the 'hedonic treadmill' and once on it, some people struggle all their lives to get off.

What about other life circumstances? Physical attractiveness is no guarantee of happiness. Thousands and thousands of people turn to cosmetic surgery to enhance their appearance in the belief that if they change their look, they will be happy. Excluding those with medically justifiable reasons for having surgery, I am referring to those who are prepared to go under the knife and alter themselves to fit some societal construct of what attractiveness is. A person may well be happy with the results immediately after surgery. Once they become accustomed to their new look they begin to take it for granted. Thoughts of surgery either stop there and they realize it wasn't their appearance that caused their unhappiness in the first place, or they find another body part to be dissatisfied with and go back to change that too. That is, assuming, they can afford it. The whole process can become addictive. So much so, the final result is that Ken or Barbie doll look that no-one finds attractive anyway.

Early in this chapter, I asked what makes you happy. Did your looks even figure in the equation? Probably not. Most naturally attractive people take their good looks for granted.

After all that, you might think I am against cosmetic surgery. I am not. I would say that if you are thinking about it, seriously consider your reasons. Don't do it if you think changing your look will bring lasting happiness. It won't. If it did, the celebrities and movie stars we hold up as being the most beautiful in our society would be in a constant state of bliss. A quick flick through the stories of any magazine or newspaper on any given day will prove quite the contrary.

How about getting married? Yes, getting married makes you happier for a short while. Studies show an increase in happiness levels lasting for about two years or so. After that they drop back to base level.

If all this sounds a little negative, the good news is we adapt to our negative circumstances too. I can testify personally to that.

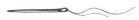

Going through the misery and uncertainty of losing a business was initially devastating, there is no denying. A few months, even weeks, later, the impact of it was much less. We adapted to our new and different circumstances.

Exceptions to this include the death of a loved one, which is an event that many people never *adapt* to. Others are permanently affected by the long term care of seriously ill relatives. Events such as losing a job or accidents of some kind might take longer but research demonstrates that, eventually, most of us adapt to even these circumstances.

So, if fifty per cent of your happiness level is determined by genetics and only ten per cent by circumstances; what about the other forty per cent

The Fun Part

Here's the fun part. forty per cent of your happiness level is determined by 'intentional activity'. That means your thoughts, your actions and your behaviours. This is exciting because all of these things can be changed. Intentional activity is where you can raise your happiness levels because what you think, what you do, and how you behave is entirely up to you. This discovery has the most amazing implications.

You are in Control

One day, during The Twilight Zone, Robin and I spent the afternoon at the hospital meeting with genetic experts about Charlotte. We'd had a trying day so decided to take the children out for dinner that night. The evening together was lively and full of fun, but try as I might, I just couldn't shake the feeling of doom. A black cloud hung over me and I knew what it was. It was a particular fear I had spent the last few months refusing to surrender to. Now, I could feel it threatening to take over and pull me into the abyss. It was a fear I needed to face. Later that night, when the children were in bed, I went to see my mother. It was the only time I ever fully gave vent to the fear that we might actually lose our precious little girl.

I gave in to despair and, like a little girl myself, broke down and wept uncontrollably at Mum's knee. She sat by the fire and I collapsed to the floor, wailing in agony and clinging on to her knees. I sunk deep down inside to the fears in the pit of my stomach, the rational and irrational, and spat them out between the sobs that racked my whole body. Mum sat quietly the whole time, listening and stroking my hair.

After a while, becoming exhausted, my sobs began to subside. Mum finally spoke. 'Come on, you've faced it now, and felt it. You've survived, you're okay. Now you can forget it. Shall I put the kettle on?' What magic there is in a cup of tea. We drank gallons of it that night and talked until the early hours.

'Face it, feel it, forget it.' Not easy. And I couldn't forget it but it was out of my system and in the open. I felt so much more able to deal with everything. That process, now known as the 'three "F"s', helped me then and has done so many times since. However, I don't recommend you try this yourself, unless you have a trusted friend, family member, or even counsellor to support you through it.

One of the things I said to Mum that night at her house was that I didn't think I would ever be happy again. Her response surprised me. It still does. Shaking her head she said to me quite firmly, 'Well, Christine, that's a decision you are going to have to make yourself.' Incredulously, I asked, 'What do you mean? A decision I have to make? You can't just decide to be happy.'

Mum was so perceptive because it turns out, yes you can. The term 'in pursuit of happiness' is a misnomer. You don't have to go looking for happiness; it's right there for the taking.

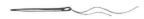

Make the decision to be happy and help yourself to it.

The problem with statistics such as the forty per cent solution is that real life isn't as neatly packaged. There is at least one other study along these lines where the percentage defining the genetic set point differs slightly. There could be others. For me, the important part of these studies is the fact that there is a large percentage of your happiness level that is determined by your own actions.

Start by deciding to change your intentional activity. Change your thoughts, your actions and behaviours, and increase your own happiness levels.

Before you can change your thoughts you have to first become aware of them (see page 43). It takes practice, and I have to warn you that when you do become aware of your thoughts, you will be amazed at how negative they are. We are believed to have around 60,000 thoughts in a day; most of them are the same thoughts as yesterday and eighty per cent of them are negative. The Buddha said:

'All that we are is the result of what we have thought. The mind is everything. What we think, we become.'

Neuroscience teaches that every thought you have produces a chemical in the brain. The chemical transmits signals to the body to allow your body to feel the thought you were thinking. So every thought is matched by a feeling in your body. If your thought is positive, the brain produces dopamine that causes you to feel uplifted or inspired. You feel good. If your thought is negative, the brain produces neuropeptides that cause you to feel upset or angry. You feel bad. The feelings, in turn, send messages back to the brain causing it to respond. You begin to think the way you are feeling. It's a cycle. If eighty per cent of what you think every day is negative, is it any wonder you are not flourishing and experiencing positive emotions most of the time?

Your thinking will start to change simply by having the intention to increase your happiness and well-being. The Conroy Concept will show you ways to make it happen.

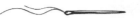

Life can be hard and bad things happen, I know. You may be unable to change what happens to you in life but, as Viktor Frankl said, you can change your attitude towards it.

You can choose to survive and thrive.

Now, it's time to have your chocolate cake and eat it.

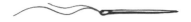

CHAPTER THREE

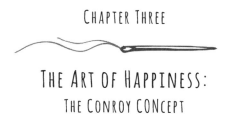

THE ART OF HAPPINESS:
THE CONROY CONCEPT

ORIGINS

The end of life came for Mum at seventy-two. I purposefully use that term, 'the end of life', because I think the word 'died' is too final. I believe there is more when we leave this world and I know Mum did too.

Given the circumstances of her cancer, Mum's passing was as good as it could have been. She had made it clear to her family that she wanted to stay at home until the end. Between us, my siblings and I made it happen. Mum lived alone but, towards the end, when she began to struggle to look after herself, a family friend moved in to help her. The rest of us arranged our visits so that she always had someone there.

I feel privileged to have been with Mum when she took her final, peaceful breath here on earth. She was at home, and comfortable in her own bed.

The previous evening to this, we, her children, sat around her bed, chatting, eating supper and drinking wine. She said goodbye to each one of us in turn. I remember thinking, 'I hope the end of my life is exactly like this.' In fact, it should be more like that for everyone. I have had many conversations with people since then and have heard dreadful stories about how their loved ones left this world. It pains me to hear such tales. For other cultures, the end of life is much more of a sacred event. It's time we learned from them and started to recognize it as such ourselves.

During an earlier visit with Mum, she started a conversation about being judgemental. She referred to a friend of hers whom she felt she had wrongly, harshly judged. That began a series of conversations we had on my visits that were some of the most honest and open we had ever had. We talked about the past but we talked about our spiritual beliefs and philosophies on life too. During this time, our relationship was finally and fully reconciled.

My mother was a strong, down to earth, practical woman. Today, I often hear myself saying, '*Mum used to say…*,' and that's followed by a nugget of wisdom that usually puts a situation into perspective, or a wrong to right. It was Mum who inspired me to start a business using my own studies and experiences to help others. It seemed only fitting when naming my business to dedicate it to her – Conroy is my mother's maiden name.

The Conroy Concept of Happiness and Well-being is a combination of over thirty years of personal development research, lessons learned through The Twilight Zone, my experiences as a coach and lecturer, and continued studies in positive psychology. It isn't complete. Like me, it's a work in progress. I am always reading and attending lectures or seminars to learn more about how to help others to make life easier, more enjoyable and fulfilling.

Throughout the Conroy Concept, I offer personal stories about cancer and illness, about the threat of losing a child and the death of loved ones. I talk about relationships and I talk about financial downfall. I use these stories to demonstrate that the Conroy Concept offers practical and effective suggestions to help you deal with whatever life issue is challenging you right now. In addition, I talk about fun and pleasure, love and friendship, and, of course, happiness and well-being.

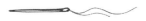

Exercises for you to try are suggested throughout the Concept. I use only those exercises that worked for us and/ or that are supported by the intensive research given to us by positive psychology. As I said in the introduction, choose only the ones that appeal to you and ignore the rest.

Part of my work is to coach people through the stages of the Concept. Similar to using a personal trainer at the gym to help you get fit and stay fit, my aim is to help you train your thoughts, mind and behaviour so that you can become happier, more resilient and more deeply satisfied with your life.

Please choose to take action. Don't let this book simply be an enjoyable read. Instead, allow it to be your kick-start to a life filled with happiness and well-being.

The Conroy Concept

The C in Concept is for Close Relationships

Your relationships are way up there at the top of the importance scale for helping you to live a fulfilling life. We are social beings and we need each other. You cannot be happy in isolation. Especially important is to nurture good relationships with those closest to you. Yet, these are often the ones we neglect the most. During our 'empire building' stage, Robin and I often worked seven days a week. I confess, we neglected relationships with friends and family. We lived in our own little world, rarely taking downtime with each other, let alone taking time to chat on the phone with anyone else. Sometimes that's all it takes to nourish a relationship – picking up the phone to say hello. Of course, these days you can use texts, which, on the upside, means it's easier to shoot off a few words to let someone know you are thinking of them. Nevertheless, a telephone call occasionally is well worth the extra effort. If, as you are reading this, someone comes to mind who you have been meaning to call – stop reading. Do it now. Pick up the phone. I will still be here when you have finished your call…

Deepening and cultivating relationships is essential to increased happiness and well-being. Here's an exercise for you to try, but before you do let me explain where it came from.

Soon after we were told that the problem with Charlotte's arm was a tumour (and not an old fracture that hadn't healed properly, which is what we had been led to believe), we sat Charlotte down to talk to her about it. Although I agreed to do the talking, I was uncertain and nervous about how to approach the conversation. Which words should I use to explain cancer, for instance, without scaring her half to death? Finally, I took a deep breath and started talking. Part way through my explanation, Charlotte excused herself to get some juice and I whispered to Robin, 'How am I doing?'

'On a scale of 1-10?' he asked. 'Twelve.'

That scaling system stuck with us. We used it for all kinds of things and eventually it evolved into this exercise. Give it a try. It's fun and it works.

EXERCISE 1:
HOW AM I DOING?

Think of someone close to you. Let's imagine it's your mother and you are the daughter. Wait until you are having a good, relaxed time together and ask her the following question:

'On a scale of 1-10, how am I doing as a daughter at the moment?'

If the answer is, for example, six, ask, 'What can I do to make it a seven?' Or, if the answer is eight, what can you do to make it nine? You get the idea.

Don't ask how to be a ten because we are none of us perfect and the effort needed to get that far might be overwhelming. In fact, if the answer is 'eight', you are actually doing exceptionally well as a daughter. Keep doing what you are doing.

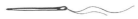

I suggested this exercise to a client when we were talking about his wife. I told him to ask her, 'On a scale of 1-10, how am I doing as a husband?' He laughed out loud telling me that, at the moment, she would say a two at most. My immediate inclination was to ask, 'What on earth makes you think only a two?' Instead, I asked him, 'So what is making you a two as opposed to a one? You must be doing something right. Let's start from there and build on it.'

The exercise should be about positives, not negatives. How to do more of what is good, as opposed to less of what is bad. Less of what is bad can easily slip into accusations and criticism, and that defeats the object.

Carried out in a light-hearted, well-intentioned way, this exercise works well within any relationship. I have even used it with my children. Although, I do remember times when, berating them for failing to do their homework or having untidy rooms, I would hear one of them mutter challengingly, 'Just ask me now how you are doing as a parent?' On other occasions I would hear somebody shouting, 'Zero! Zero!' all over the house. They would usually be laughing as they went, but the message was loud and clear. They were upset about something.

Remember to wait for the right moment and keep the conversation light and positive. You might be surprised by what you learn. What will take you up to the next level? Asking the question alone will improve your relationship. It demonstrates that you want to be better, which shows how much you care. The important thing then is to try to act on the answer given.

Robin and I have been together for over thirty years and we continue to do this exercise learning something different every time.

If you don't feel you can ask this of someone in person, ask yourself what you think they (whomever it is you choose) would answer. Think about that person right now. Ask yourself the question... Write down your own answers and start to act on them.

Social support from family and friends is so necessary to well-

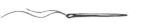
being. Mum used to say, 'You are lucky to have a handful of true friends during a lifetime.' How true those words are.

You certainly find out who your true friends are when you are in trouble. Or, should I say, who are not your friends. It's almost a cliché to say that people cross the road when they see you coming, but some people do. If you are ever tempted to do that because you spot someone ahead whom you know is ill or has had a recent bereavement, I beg you to reconsider. It happened to us more than once and it was shocking and hurtful.

A bewildering incident happened to me when Charlotte was recovering from the amputation of her arm. Few people knew the details of what was happening to her but the amputation was, obviously, common knowledge in the community.

Out shopping one day, I literally bumped into two people who knew Charlotte well. I greeted them and started a conversation. Before long I began to realize that they were not going to ask how we were, or even mention what had happened. Shifting from one leg to another and looking everywhere but straight at me, they were obviously itching to move on. They were so painfully uncomfortable, it was embarrassing. I released them by saying, 'Anyway, must dash, I have to be somewhere.' I hurried away, almost in tears. Within seconds of that horrible meeting, I met a mum from Charlotte's school. This was a lady I didn't know very well at all. By contrast, she rushed up to me and immediately asked, 'How is Charlotte?' She invited me for a coffee, but only if I felt like talking. I did. There were no tears, I didn't break down. I talked, she listened. That's all. Our paths didn't cross much after that and we didn't speak properly again. She will never know how much that coffee, on that day, meant to me. Well, she might do now.

Without explanation, some people never contacted us again. Others waited until we were out of The Twilight Zone before speaking to us. We found it bizarre the way different people reacted in totally unexpected ways.

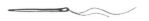

It was my perceptive local doctor who pointed out to me that our experience with Charlotte was forcing our friends to face their own worst fears – the death of one of their children. Some people simply couldn't handle it. I understand that now. I didn't at the time.

Thankfully, we did have friends who stayed right beside us for the long haul and we appreciate them so much. Similarly, we were thankful for friendships that were rekindled during that time. An army of others, from complete strangers to customers and business colleagues, went out of their way to comfort us. That kind of support is a huge lift to the spirit. It makes such a difference to know you are not alone.

I understand it isn't always easy but if you know someone is in need, go with your instinct and reach out to them. People sometimes tell me, 'But I feel so bad and I just don't know what to say.' Well that's a start, right there. Turn up and say, 'I don't know what to say.'

Often there is nothing to say. In any case, your actions will speak much louder than anything you could say. If people see you struggling but showing up anyway, it gives them permission to do the same. Don't allow being unsure of what to say stop you. You will be so pleased you made the effort and it will strengthen and deepen your relationship.

The opposite of this is those people who cannot share your good fortune. Sometimes you find out who are not your friends when things are going well for you. Perhaps you have achieved something your friend hasn't yet managed and they just can't be happy for you. It happens.

We learned from all of this that there are times when you have to put your own feelings aside. It might be uncomfortable at first but it won't be for long. You never know, you might need the favour returned sometime. It says in the Bible:

'Therefore all things whatsoever ye would that men should do to you, do ye even so to them.'

In other words, treat others the way you would like to be treated yourself.

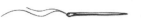

I love the poem 'The Invitation' by Oriah Mountain Dreamer and I include two verses of it here. She says:

It doesn't interest me what planets are squaring your moon.
I want to know if you have touched the centre of your own sorrow,
if you have been opened by life's betrayals or have become shrivelled
and closed from fear of further pain. I want to know if you can sit with pain,
mine or your own, without moving to hide it or fade it or fix it.

And then she goes on:

I want to know if you can be with joy, mine or your own,
if you can dance with wildness and let the ecstasy fill you...

Wonderful sentiments so eloquently expressed. I urge you to read the rest of the poem, 'The Invitation' and the book about its origins and meanings.

My family and I now know for certain that if disaster strikes again we are surrounded by true friends who will stay to support us and we them. Without trusted people around us, we are lost.

The thirteenth century Christian philosopher St Thomas Aquinas said, 'There is nothing on this earth to be prized more than true friendship.'

Go and ask someone, 'On a scale of 1-10, how am I doing as a friend?'

THE O IN CONCEPT IS FOR OUTCOME

Being outcome-focused and goal-oriented. There is a direct link between pursuing goals and happiness.

Whenever we faced bad news about Charlotte, my mum or my sister, the question I always asked was, 'What is the worst case

scenario?' When asking a question like that on behalf of someone else, be sure they want to know the answer too. Some people don't want that kind of information and that has to be respected. I felt I needed to be prepared for whatever we might have to deal with, no matter how bad. That way, I would be better equipped to support whomever we were discussing. The down-side to that is that I wasted much of my time agonizing over things that might happen but rarely did. That way of thinking didn't help any of us. Instead, I started asking, 'What's the best we can hope for here?' And that's what we tried to aim for. That didn't always work either.

Of course, the ideal solution, in this situation, is to prepare for the worst and hope for the best. Unfortunately, like many of these 'wise' solutions, it is much easier said than done. We tried most of the time.

Being able to focus on the best possible outcome is easier if you have emotional support. Robin and I promised each other that if we were feeling negative in any way, we would say so. There were many times when we had to talk each other out of fear and into hope. Sometimes there was no positive outcome. Mum was terminally ill and we had to accept that. After that, the best outcome was that the life she had remaining be as good as it could possibly be. Additionally, that meant that she leave this world pain-free and at peace. She did.

Robin and I had to reach our lowest point where we had lost almost everything before we realized that being outcome-oriented didn't only apply when dealing with illness. It might be strange that you should expect it to, but the rest of life does not stop when cancer comes to call. There are still other life issues to deal with. At that time, we lived our lives fighting fires that were out of control. We simply reacted to everything being thrown at us. The business was going down, we had no income and even our savings had gone.

It was Christmas Eve. We had been relying on a colleague who owed us a considerable amount of money to pay it back. He didn't and he wasn't returning our calls.

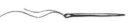

Father Christmas wasn't coming to our house that year…

Oh, yes he was.

We hunted our colleague down and accepted as much as he could afford towards payment of his loan, and at teatime we went shopping. We were up all through the night wrapping gifts, preparing for Christmas and talking. Together on that Christmas Eve we made the conscious decision to change our attitudes. We didn't know what the future held for our family but we knew we had to live now. We would do everything in our power for our daughter but if she was going to leave this world sooner rather than later, so be it. That was out of our control. What we could ensure was that she and the boys enjoyed what time we had left together. We were going to make the most of our lives.

One night during the following week, after we put the children to bed, Robin and I sat down with pen and paper. We asked ourselves what we really wanted out of life. Not what we thought we should want. What did we really want? What would be the absolute best outcome of our situation for our family? Happiness and well-being? What did that mean for us?

We imagined where we wanted to be two years, five years and ten years down the line. We decided we wanted what we had before. We loved the business we were in but it needed to be on a much smaller scale. We didn't want a huge workforce to be responsible for and concerned about. We wanted to work together but divide our time equally so that we both cared for the children, without nannies. On a lighter note, Robin wanted to be able to coach American football and have his sons play the game. I wanted to study Art and Design History. We both visualized celebrating our daughter's twenty-first birthday.

That day during the Christmas holidays, we started to see a little sunshine poking through the clouds. A brighter day dawning – the day we started to take control of our lives.

Now you might think all this a tad unrealistic given our

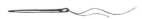

situation. We were flexible. We decided if we shoot for the moon and miss, we would, at least, gather some stars along the way. Once we had our overall visions, we started to set goals. Even now, all these years later, we regularly go away for the weekend and spend time revisiting our goals. We assess our current situation and decide what we want to do next. Some goals are added and others adapted. It ensures that we both still want the same things and are heading in the same direction.

I use the same approach with others. Philip has been in business for over twenty years. He owns a shop selling sofas and occasional furniture. Originally, he came to me because business wasn't good and he felt it might be time for a change. He had no enthusiasm for his work. He had tried everything to increase sales and worried about what would happen if things didn't improve soon. People sometimes get stuck in the problem. They ruminate over it, dissect it, and try to establish the causes of it. Often they can't see beyond the problem apart from its negative consequences.

We shifted Philip's thinking by talking about what his business would look like if he had all the customers he needed. How would he feel? What difference would it make to him? I asked if his business had ever been that good, and he said it had. His energy changed when he talked about it. It was clear that the enthusiasm he had for his business when he first started out was still there. He just needed to be reminded of it. We talked about what he had done in the past that made business so good, and we discussed the current resources he could use to help him now.

Eventually, Philip decided to develop the public relations side of his business. Once he had made that decision there was no stopping him. He came up with all kinds of ideas about what he wanted to do. What happened here, with a gentle push from me, is Philip changed his way of thinking. I believe that you are the expert in your own life. The job of a coach is to help you discover your own answers, which are always there if you dig deep enough. Once

Philip changed his thinking and decided on the outcome he wanted, he started to set goals.

GOAL SETTING

Having goals creates something to aim for and gives a sense of meaning and purpose. Your goals will motivate you and give you direction. In order to achieve something, you first have to know what you want. You don't start that journey in a taxi without knowing your destination. Okay, occasionally, it might be fun to set out and see where the wind takes you. If you live your whole life that way, you will simply drift and end up going nowhere.

Knowing what you want is often the most difficult step. The number of my students who had no idea what they wanted to do greatly concerned me. They were at university because that's what was expected of them. After that, they had no idea. Another 'off curriculum' class took place on goal setting. My advice to them, as to my own teenagers, was 'design your life'. My students enjoyed the following exercise. It might help you.

EXERCISE 2:
FUTURE YOU

Close your eyes and take a few long, deep breaths. Let the out-breath be slightly longer than the in-breath. This has a calming effect. Let go and relax your body. Imagine that you are walking down a street in your town ten years from now. You are relaxed and content with life. You have achieved everything you have ever wanted. You turn a corner and bump straight into someone you haven't seen since your school days. They say, 'Wow! You look fantastic. What are you doing these days?'

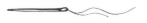

> Choose from one of the following and tell them all the things you have achieved in that area. Let your imagine run without limitation:
>
> • Career
> • Personal
> • Spiritual
> • Finance
> • Health
> • Family

When you have the time, go through the process in all of these areas and write down your answers. Let your answers form the overall vision for your life. If you can't imagine ten years, try five, or two, but give it your full attention. It doesn't matter what might happen down the line. You start off with an overall plan that will no doubt change and grow as you do and that's okay – your plan is not set in stone. Now you can start to set both short and long term goals with your plan or vision in mind.

When setting goals, try not to think too much about how you are going to achieve them all. Each time you achieve one of your short term goals you will have learned something more about yourself or your field than you knew before. You will grow as you move forward. By the time you come to your long term goals, you will have acquired the information you need along the way. Achieving goals is not only about the goal itself, but also about how you develop personally in their pursuit.

Most people give more consideration to their annual holiday than they do to their lives. I love what Brian Tracy says, 'Only three per cent of adults have clearly written down goals… and everyone else works for them.'

Of course, goal setting is not for students alone. C.S. Lewis said, 'You are never too old to set a new goal or dream a new dream.' I agree.

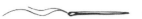

Here's how to do it:

EXERCISE 3:
GOAL SETTING

1) Decide on your goal.
2) Make it specific and realistic. Write it down.
3) Give your goal an achievable deadline.
4) Visualize the outcome.
5) Break it down into manageable action steps.
6) Take action.
7) Acknowledge each small achievement you make towards your goal.
8) Celebrate success.

Remember, a goal is just a dream if you ignore step six.

For example:

'I feel I am overweight at the moment and could look better. I want to lose the excess weight.' Taking that through the goal setting process, my overall vision is to look and feel the best I can.

1) The goal: To lose weight.
2) I write down: I am 7 lb. lighter.

Goals are always better written in the present tense. This is something I have only recently discovered myself. It makes the goal more believable and motivates the right action.

3) I also write down: It is now June 30th (eight weeks from now) and I am 7 lb lighter.

I have calculated here to lose one pound a week, with one week's grace built in where I don't lose any weight at all. I consider this to be realistic weight loss.

4) I close my eyes, relax, and visualize the following scene: I am entering a restaurant wearing my gorgeous red dress (the one I don't fit into at the moment). I look fantastic. As I walk in the room, people stop what they are doing to look at me. Everyone starts to applaud as I walk through the restaurant to my table. I feel fabulous.

Be as outrageous as you like with this step. Make it fun. 'Visualize' is another word for 'imagine', except that you don't just see yourself in your mind, you also imagine how you feel. How will you feel when your goal is achieved? The more emotional the better.

5) Research healthy eating plan. Throw out or give away all chocolate, biscuits, cakes and other unhealthy food. Make a meal plan. Grocery shop for healthy foods.
6) I decide on a healthy eating plan.
7) Once a week I check my weight loss and reward myself for every pound I lose (not with chocolate or cake).
8) Go to restaurant wearing my red dress.

A note about visualization. It is also known as mental imagery or rehearsal and has been used by athletes for years. When you visualize, new neural pathways are created in your brain as if you had actually performed the action. The brain cannot distinguish between the imagined and the actual event. In sport, it has been demonstrated to improve performance as though the athlete has been physically practising. In terms of use for personal development and, in this case, goal setting, it helps to create belief first in the subconscious mind, which then comes through to the conscious mind and motivates the right action to achieve. As the saying goes

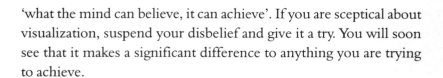
'what the mind can believe, it can achieve'. If you are sceptical about visualization, suspend your disbelief and give it a try. You will soon see that it makes a significant difference to anything you are trying to achieve.

THE N IN CONCEPT IS FOR NOW

Referring to mindfulness. Living in the present moment. Living Now. After all that consideration of the future and setting goals, I am now strongly urging you to live in the moment. This is not a contradiction. Once you have an overall plan for the rest of your life and have set goals and action steps, start living in the present. Work towards your goals but enjoy the process along the way. Being present means being fully engaged in the moment and being open and curious about it, without distractions.

I mentioned that during The Twilight Zone, I had to stop asking what would be the worst case scenario of a situation? I found myself constantly worrying about events that only might happen. In everyday life, negative 'self-talk' is what most of us engage in, albeit about less dramatic situations. That little voice in your head, running along, mostly unnoticed, offering up negative 'what ifs?' all the time. What if… I don't get that job? What if… they don't like me? What if… I can't afford it? What if… I can't do it? And, so on. Mark Twain said, 'I've had thousands of problems in my life – most of which have never actually happened.' My first question in any situation now is, 'What are the facts?' or 'What do you know be true, right now, at this moment?' You can only work with what you know now. If the facts include that in a few days' time, or sometime in the future, a particular thing is going to happen, then you can work to prepare for it. Other than that, consider only the known facts of the present situation. That means no more unnecessary worrying. Are you ready for that?

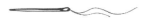

It requires becoming more aware of your thinking and being brutally honest with yourself. If change is to happen, the desire or, in my case, the need to change has to be strong enough. Believe it or not, worrying is a habit, even an addiction that some people don't want to overcome. You might find that this aspect of living in the Now is the most difficult to master – I did. All I can say is that practice really does make perfect. I don't manage to do this all the time, although I can honestly say, I do it most of the time. Coaching can help.

Let's assume for a minute that you want to overcome unnecessary worrying and you don't have a personal coach to help you. How do you do it?

The first step is to recognize when you are doing it. Become conscious of your negative thinking. The way to do that is to check in on how you are feeling. As mentioned in the science part of this book, all of your thoughts have corresponding feelings. I feel my thoughts in my tummy. When I am happy or excited, I get a feeling like little fluttering butterflies there. If I'm exceptionally lucky, the butterflies escape and flutter all around my body, which is wonderful. When I am hurt, anxious or worried, I get what I call a pit in my stomach. It feels a bit like a brick lodged there. Depending on the severity of the situation, that brick weighs heavy. Sometimes it smoulders, then it burns. The burning brick is when I get pain. How do you feel your thoughts? You will know. Being present with your feelings means checking in with them. Ask yourself: How am I feeling right now? Your days might be so busy that you forget to do this until bedtime. If that's the case you need to set up triggers. Each time I get a stop light when I'm out in the car, I check how I'm feeling. I have a client who sets a timer on his computer at work to go off every two hours to remind him. Someone else uses their phone. It only takes a second to do and after a while it will become second nature. If you check in and, yes, you have a pit in your stomach, or the equivalent, ask yourself what are you thinking about?

STOP 'THINGING'

You need to beware of the three 'ings':

1) Ruminating – churning the same thing over and over
2) Imagining – what if?
3) Exaggerating – making something worse than it is

Once you recognize yourself doing any of the three things that I call 'thinging', you are on your way to stopping it. Say to yourself, 'Christine (your name, of course), you're doing it again.' Bring your full attention back to wherever you are. Concentrate on what you are actually doing at that time. Use your senses to ground you in the moment. What can you see, feel, hear, and even smell?

The following is an example of all three 'ings' happening to one person: Shirley is another long-time business owner. Each year she ran up a personal tax bill, which she paid the following year from the profits her business made. She never bothered to put money away as she earned it because the profits had always been there.

The inevitable happened and Shirley found that her business had suffered in the recession. There was no money to pay her tax bill. She had never been in this position before and was distraught. She kept asking herself how she could be so stupid. The constant reminders and telephone calls from the Inland Revenue went ignored because Shirley saw no way to pay the debt. She continued to worry (ruminating). Her concerns ranged from losing her business to being 'clapped in irons' (imagining). Worrying about the lack of funds wasn't doing anything to solve the situation.

The worrying started to adversely affect her business decisions and her relationship with her partner, who was unaware of the situation. Shirley felt that if her partner knew she owed thousands and thousands (exaggerating) to the Inland Revenue, he would think

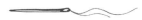

her foolish. This situation was clearly having a huge effect on her life and so it became the focus of our session.

As I considered how best to help her change her way of thinking, my phone rang. Unusually, I had forgotten to unplug. It was one of those irritating recorded messages telling me that I could claim back the personal insurance if I had taken out loans. I must have complained about it because Shirley erupted into a tirade of abuse about this type of call, which she got all the time. She went on to say how she immediately slams the phone down if she answers, only to find herself speaking to a machine. She didn't need reminding that she couldn't take out another loan to help pay her tax bill. 'So you have taken out loans in the past?' I asked. 'Well, yes...' she answered. That was her 'aha' moment, right there.

Shirley didn't wait for another annoying call but contacted the claims company immediately. Eventually, she received the compensation, which was almost enough to cover her tax bill. She had allowed the three 'ings' to get in the way of her solution.

The Filing Cabinet

If you are not 'thinging' but have a genuine concern, file it until you have the opportunity to address it properly. The filing system process was given to me by my sister, Pat, who is an expert at it.

Quite simply, imagine a filing cabinet in your mind, open up a drawer and drop in your worry. Tell yourself you are not ignoring it, you are putting it away until the time is right to do something about it. Now bring your attention back to where you are and what you are doing and focus on that instead. At a suitable time, retrieve your concern from the filing cabinet. Consider the issue and apply the O or Outcome of the Concept. Ask yourself, 'What's the best possible outcome for me in this situation?' Make it a goal. Work

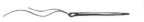

back from there and create the action steps you think will help you reach that conclusion. Then take action. Even though you might never reach that perfect conclusion, you will approach your problem in the right frame of mind and have a much better chance of success.

Pat employs the 'filing cabinet' system whenever she has to wait for results of serious tests. The waiting in these situations is often unbearable. If she has tests on Monday and has to wait until Friday for results, she files the problem, telling herself she will open it up on Thursday night. She explains that each time the thought of the results pops into her mind, she takes a few minutes to close her eyes, take a few deep breaths, and imagines filing it again. Don't be fooled by the simplicity of the filing cabinet; it works.

MEDITATION

When I first discovered meditation over twenty-five years ago, I struggled with it. I played with it really, only remembering to try it occasionally. It was when I was introduced to yoga that I truly began a meditation practice. Practising yoga itself slowed down my body and mind in preparation to sit in meditation. It wasn't long before I began to feel a strong sense of peace after sitting that stayed with me long after the meditation. That calm and peaceful feeling continues to bring me back.

You don't have to do yoga to practise meditation, nor do you need to do anything complicated. If you have never meditated before, try this:

EXERCISE 4:
MEDITATION

Sit crossed legged on the floor with a cushion under your bottom, if necessary. You can sit upright on a chair with your feet on the ground if that's more comfortable. Put your hands on your tummy so that when you breathe in through your nose, you can feel your tummy rise, like a balloon blowing up. When you exhale, your tummy comes back down. That's the way to breathe – through your tummy. Again, let the out-breath be slightly longer than the in-breath. Once you have perfected the breathing, rest your hands on your lap and close your eyes. Take one or two long, deep breaths to relax and let your shoulders drop. Breathe in and start to count your out-breaths – One, breathe in, breathe out – Two, and so on. Focus totally on your breath; feel it come in and go out. Count to four then go back to one and start the process again.

Your mind will wander. The key is to be aware of the thoughts that appear, acknowledge them, and let them go. If you can, detach from your thoughts, watch them without becoming lost in them. Let the thoughts pass by, then gently come back to the breath and the counting. It's an easy way to start a meditation practice. For a free download of this meditation, go to my website, www.ChristineLConroy.com/meditation. It is designed as an introduction to get you strated with meditation.

Never think you are too busy or have too much to think about to sit still for a while. Those times are precisely when you need to do it. You will find that after meditation, your thinking is clearer and much sharper than before. As is the case with being mindful and living in the moment, meditation is also about focussed attention. You can do it anywhere at any time, even for a few minutes at your desk at lunchtime, for example. When I am about to speak to an audience, I practise this meditation for about ten minutes beforehand. It helps with nerves and keeps me grounded in the present moment.

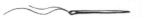

I like to add a spiritual element to my meditation and create a ritual out of my practice but it isn't necessary to do so.

The past has gone and the future hasn't happened yet. You only have right now. Life is happening in this moment – be present with it. Live Now.

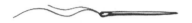

CHAPTER FOUR

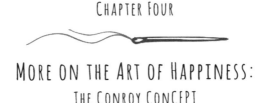

MORE ON THE ART OF HAPPINESS:
THE CONROY CONCEPT

Before we move on, take a long deep inhale of breath and exhale slowly. And again. Have the intention to take control of your own happiness. Be right here with me in this moment as we explore the next part of the Conroy Concept.

THE SECOND C IN CONCEPT IS FOR CONTRIBUTION

Most of us want to feel that we contribute to the greater good and hopefully make a difference in the world. It gives us purpose and meaning. Without that, our lives can feel empty. I believe most of us do contribute in our own ways.

To contribute means to give something in order to achieve something. You do that on a daily basis when you go to work in your particular field. The fact that you are financially rewarded for your labours doesn't make what you do any less of a contribution. If you are a parent, the biggest single contribution you can make to the greater good is to teach your children how to become good citizens. If everyone did that, we would know for sure that when we leave this world, it will be a better place than we found it. A simple, idealistic thing to say? Perhaps. But we have to start somewhere and home is a good place.

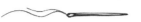

In 2012 the world's population hit seven billion. That's a lot of people sharing the earth. We can't afford to live looking out only for ourselves and taking what we need without giving something back. The majority of us are beginning to understand that. In addition to being altruistic, it really is true that by helping others you will help yourself. Helping others makes you feel good about yourself, doesn't it? If you have any doubts about that, try this exercise:

EXERCISE 5:
BE KIND

Think of three kind things you could do for three different people today. Small things such as pay for your friend's coffee at lunchtime, go out of your way to help a co-worker, offer to carry someone's bags, or let someone go before you in traffic. I don't mean to be patronizing here. I'm sure you automatically do these things anyway. This exercise is about doing these things consciously. Be totally aware of what you are doing. Notice how the other person reacts to you. Notice, especially, how it makes you feel. I guarantee you will feel a little lift in your mood.

I am not suggesting that you should be helping others purely for selfish reasons. The thing about these acts is that they have a ripple effect. By helping someone else, you cheer them up. They are much more likely to feel charitable towards the next person they meet. By helping them, your mood is lifted and you, too, will carry the mood over. Goodwill spreads. You have contributed by making someone else's day that little bit better and they go on to do the same.

You can, of course, help others in bigger ways. One option is to volunteer your time or services. Volunteering lifts your mood but is also associated with enhanced feelings of personal control, self-esteem and confidence. These aspects of personality are the exact same ones that you will need to draw on in order to meet life's

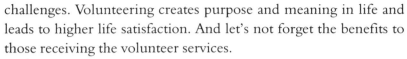

challenges. Volunteering creates purpose and meaning in life and leads to higher life satisfaction. And let's not forget the benefits to those receiving the volunteer services.

Investigate the possibilities for yourself. Find a way to do it that captures your imagination. You will be far more effective as a volunteer if you choose to do something because you enjoy it rather than because you feel you ought to. Don't feel you need to be like Mother Theresa. One of the things I do is to volunteer at the local art gallery. It might not be helping the sick or the homeless but being able to make someone's day that little bit more enjoyable is a fantastic feeling. It gives me great pleasure to know that I contribute to the visitor's enjoyment.

You might feel able to mentor a young person. Robin joined a mentoring scheme in our town. His mentees have been aged between eleven and sixteen years old. No matter how old you are, you are ahead of somebody else in terms of experience. There could be a young person out there who would benefit enormously from your life expertise. Just one hour a week makes such a difference to a person who possibly has nobody else to talk to. Robin would tell you himself that the mentoring experience changed his whole way of thinking about the world. I think most towns have schemes operating like this. If your town doesn't, maybe you could start one.

My sons love sport. You guessed it. They play American football. Both have been involved in setting up community football teams and coaching the game. Sport, in general, is a fantastic way of bringing people together, especially in areas where children have no other recreational facilities. American football is particularly good because even those who are less athletic can play the game. Young people who have never had the experience of being part of a team before can take part.

Volunteering has given my children more understanding of those less fortunate than themselves. This resulted in them being more compassionate for others and more appreciative of what they have in their own lives.

Think about your own particular strengths and how they can best be put to use in a volunteering situation.

The charity Depression Alliance even reports that volunteering does, in fact, help to combat depression. Volunteering is a 'win-win situation.'

The E in CONCEPT is for Exercise

E is about exercise, sports, *and* health. I do hope you are not rolling your eyes at the mention of exercise. I say that because I recently gave a speech where I spoke of exercise being the elixir of youth. A large section of the audience audibly groaned. 'We know we need to exercise,' they said. Strangely, when I asked for a show of hands of how many people actually exercised on a daily basis, few hands went up. Common sense but not common practice, it would seem. Sometimes we don't need to learn new information as much as to be reminded of what we already know.

According to BUPA, the largest private medical health insurers in the UK, people who live active lives are less likely to be ill and are more likely to live longer. In case you do need to be reminded, here are a few of the possible physical benefits of exercise.

It can help to reduce the risk of heart disease and stroke, reduce blood pressure and cholesterol levels, reduce the risk of back pain, help prevent osteoporosis, and help your joints remain supple and your spine flexible. Some studies show it can even prevent certain cancers. All this, in addition to helping to maintain your weight, tone your muscles, and keep you looking great. The research couldn't be any clearer. You need to get moving and keep moving. However, what interests me the most is exercise and your mental well-being.

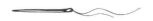

Almost every evening during The Twilight Zone I would disappear at six o'clock to go to work out. It became routine. Friends and family soon stopped contacting me during that time because they knew I would be unavailable. Each day, I chose yoga, weight training or aerobics and exercised for about an hour. Mostly, I went undisturbed but if the kids came in, they joined in. Some days it was such an enormous effort to start. I used to talk myself into it by telling myself, 'I'll just do ten minutes, maybe twenty.' I always went the full hour. The hardest part is getting started. The certainty of feeling wonderful once I had finished pushed me on. I always came out of that room feeling so much more energized than going in, and much more able to cope with the day's challenges. I don't work out every day any more but I do exercise regularly. It always lifts my mood.

As I understand it, exercise increases the body's feel good hormones, such as endorphins, and decreases stress hormones, such as cortisol. Current thinking is that thirty minutes of moderately vigorous exercise at least three times a week will do the trick. I would say five times a week with two days off. See what works for you.

EXERCISE 6:
EXERCISE

If you travel by bus, get off a few stops before you need to and briskly walk the rest of the way. I like to walk listening to upbeat music to keep my pace fast enough to get me slightly out of breath. If you can manage to do that even three times a week, you will start to feel a difference. Slowly increase your walking time. Swimming, dancing, or anything that gets you out of breath is aerobic. Yoga is relaxing because the slow and precise movements force you to concentrate on your body and therefore slows down your thinking. Furthermore, it stretches out muscles tensed through anxiety or stress accumulated during the day.

However, depending on the type of yoga you choose, it can also be aerobic and strengthening. Weight training strengthens and tones muscles. In addition, it helps to keep bones strong and healthy, which is important for women going through, and after, the menopause.

So many studies support the idea that exercise increases well-being. Ignore them at your peril. If you don't already exercise regularly, please start. You can build up to a workout class or even take up an adventure sport. Choose something you will enjoy and, if possible, do it with a friend who will encourage you at times when you feel less inclined. Of course, you must be sure to consult with your primary caregiver before starting any exercise programme.

Good health is vital to your well-being. You must pay particularly close attention to your own health when you are going through a crisis. Even more so if you are responsible for the care of somebody else. Ironically, it is often at these times when you are likely to forget about your own needs. If you are going to survive a crisis of any kind or be of any help to others, you need to be 'firing on all cylinders' or performing at your absolute best. You will find it hard to be your best if you are dogged by ill health.

I confess that there are two important pieces of health advice that I find difficult to follow. They are to drink eight glasses of water a day, and to get at least eight hours of sleep. One keeps your body hydrated, the other ensures it is well rested. These two things alone help to keep your body working at optimal levels. I struggle to drink so much water. I was, therefore, interested in a recent study that says tea and coffee are equally as effective at hydrating the body. An Australian researcher says that tea and coffee can be included as part of your eight glasses of fluid per day. I would normally wait to see other corroborating research before considering changing my behaviour to suit. In this case however, although I will continue to

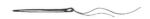

try to drink more water, I won't feel so guilty anymore about drinking so much tea.

My mother used to say, 'You can deal with most things if you have had a good night's sleep.' Unfortunately, during the night is the worst time for 'thinging' (ruminating, imagining, and exaggerating), mentioned in the last chapter. Try the following:

- Check your environment. Try to keep computers and other electronic gizmos out of your bedroom. Your sleeping area needs to be peaceful and designed to promote rest.
- As far as possible try to prevent anything waking you once you have fallen asleep. So, if you tend to use the bathroom in the middle of the night, don't drink after a certain time during the evening.
- Don't eat anything that is likely to cause indigestion and don't eat too late in the evening.
- Wear an eye mask to block out all the light.
- Close your bedroom door to keep out noise.
- Don't read scary books or watch disturbing films before going to bed.
- Try a nice warm bath before retiring and use lavender essential oil on your pillow to calm you.
- Practise the gratitude exercise (see page 82). Immediately before you go to sleep is a good time to do it.

EXERCISE 7:
BANISH NIGHT-TIME 'THINGING'

If you do wake in the night and you are unable to stop 'thinging', here is a more intense version of the filing cabinet exercise that will help.

Have a pen and paper by your bed in readiness. Accept the negative thoughts, don't fight them. Sit up, take your pen and paper and start

writing. This should be automatic free-flowing writing – literally empty your thoughts from your head on to the paper. Only you will see what you write so there is no need to censor yourself. Keep writing and if the same thoughts repeat themselves, keep writing them down. Carry on with this until there is nothing left to say. Eventually, you will stop writing. Put the paper by your bed and tell yourself you will deal with the thoughts in the morning. Mentally repeat the gratitude exercise until you go to sleep.

When those people who have done this exercise read in the morning what they thought about during the night, they are often shocked, but mostly embarrassed. Embarrassed because of the high level of 'thinging' in their thoughts, especially imagining and exaggerating. That's what the night time does to your thinking. The beauty of this exercise is what happens on consequent sleepless nights. You become almost immediately conscious that your thoughts are playing tricks on you and it takes less and less time to get them out of your head altogether. Nonetheless, it takes some practice, so stick with it.

THE P IN CONCEPT IS FOR PLEASURE

Pleasure and fun. I am going to start this section with a lovely exercise for you. It should take about ten minutes to do and you will need pen and paper.

EXERCISE 8:
DIGGING FOR PLEASURE

I would like you to make a list of ten things that give you pleasure. You

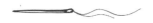

shouldn't need to think too hard about this but dig deep if you have to. I don't want you to stop until you have ten items on your list. Your items don't have to be big things. For example, and in no particular order, here are ten pleasurable things of mine.

1) **Food**. I love good food. Fortunately for me, Robin loves to cook. I especially love oysters accompanied by a small glass of smooth black velvet, (Guinness and Champagne). Rich, dark, 85% cocoa chocolate is another favourite. Of course, they are occasional treats. I also like broccoli (I know, but it is so good for you), stir fries, and any dish with chicken. On the very odd occasion, I love good old fashioned fish and chips. I could go on.

2) **White flowers**. Cut flowers in the house, of any kind, always cheer me. However, I love to fill the house with white flowers. There is a beautiful simplicity and purity to white flowers that I adore.

3) **Good design**. Most of my working life has been involved with creating good design. From designing furniture to improve the lifestyles of clients to designing programmes to help increase their happiness and well-being. Good design can change the world.

4) **Dry stone walls**. This is weird, so I have been told. Even more so when I say I prefer them wet. I love wet, dry stone walls (I smile as I write).

5) **Films**. I love the whole cinema experience. I always feel a flutter of excitement when the lights go down. I even enjoy bad films. I don't watch horror movies or those carrying an 18 certificate but, other than that, I will watch anything.

6) **Books**. I don't often read novels. In saying that, I have a reliable source for fiction recommendations. If I get a suggestion, I make the effort and always enjoy it. On the other hand, I constantly have a personal or spiritual development book on the go.

7) **Going to the hairdresser**. At my hair salon they spend time massaging your head during the hair wash, offer a glass of wine should you feel like it, and notice when you want to talk and when you don't. All in addition to turning you out of the salon looking fabulous. It's a real treat.

8) **Art.** My first degree is in Art and Design History. Such a vast subject; there is always something new to learn or see. My taste is eclectic. Often, it's the story behind the artwork that interests me more than the final creation. I love to visit art galleries.

9) **Silk sheets.** I have only recently discovered the joys of sleeping in silk. It truly is like sleeping in a cloud. Definitely worth paying the extra for or putting on your birthday or Christmas list.

10) **Family dinners.** Our children have now left home and live in various parts of the country, which makes it even more enjoyable when we do manage to eat together. Of course, it could never happen as often as I would like.

Those are ten things that give me pleasure. There are many, many more. You should now have your own list. All I want you to do is choose two of the better ones and schedule them into your diary this week. That's it. Put them in your diary because, if you are anything like me, if it isn't in your diary – it won't get done. Do not be tempted to ignore them at the scheduled time because you think you have other, more important things to do. There is no-one more important than you. Which is especially true if you spend time caring for others.

Moments of pleasure, little and often, will sustain and inspire you. Knowing that after a busy day you have scheduled time to sit down and read a great book is very motivational. Make it your business to find these little things that give you pleasure and add them to your list. Choose a different, small one on a daily basis and schedule two or three big ones over the week.

During tough times, the smallest of things gave me something to look forward to. The mere thought of a half hour to myself, soaking in a lovely, hot bath, for example, surrounded by scented candles was relaxing. Savouring a glass of something special and, on

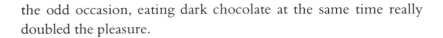

the odd occasion, eating dark chocolate at the same time really doubled the pleasure.

FUN

Vital to survival, let alone to well-being, is a sense of humour. My whole family is blessed with an easy humour that has helped us to float through some otherwise devastating times. Imagine this, if you will. I was sitting on a chair beside Charlotte in her hospital bed. She had just had the operation to remove her arm and was still sleeping from the anaesthetic. Previously, we had consulted with medical staff and counsellors about how best to help Charlotte through this traumatic time. Again, we felt anxious to get it right. I had been advised to sit on the opposite side of the amputation because Charlotte wouldn't want to look that way. I was uncomfortable with that, it felt counter-intuitive to me. So, here I was, sitting, engrossed in my own thoughts, on the same side as the amputated arm waiting for her to wake up.

In the bed opposite to Charlotte lay a stunning Indian teenage girl with enormous brown eyes and lustrous long dark hair. I will call her Elisha. Elisha spoke little English and, apparently, had severe learning difficulties. Her condition included a nervous or muscular disorder of some kind that often caused her limbs to be rigid and stiff.

Every morning Elisha was taken in a wheelchair to a meeting point outside the hospital and collected to be taken to a special school for the day. On this morning, the nurses arrived late to dress her ready for school. They were in a hurry. I was watching absent-mindedly.

My attention caught when I heard one of the nurses cursing and muttering under her breath. In order to get Elisha into the wheelchair, the nurses had to fit her with a kind of bib or harness that enabled them to fasten her safely into the chair. They were struggling. Both nurses were puffing and blowing, quickly trying to dress Elisha and put on the bib.

Watching this made me smile. It reminded me of trying to dress my children when they were small. Happy to stay in pyjamas all day, they would be purposefully uncooperative. It was often hard work.

Elisha's arm stiffened right at the moment the nurses were trying to bend it to put it through the sleeve. Her legs did the same. I started giggling. Elisha saw me and looked at me with such a knowing and mischievous glint in her eye, I felt certain she was in complete control of what she was doing. I laughed, even more. The nurses saw me laughing and started to laugh too.

They continued to struggle, stopping occasionally to take a breath. At long last they managed to lift Elisha into the chair. Next, I heard, 'Ah (bleep). The (bleep) bib's on upside down. We're gonna have to get her back on the bed and (bleep) do it all again.' That was more than I could bear. I laughed out loud and continued to laugh until tears were rolling down my face. The nurses and Elisha also surrendered and collapsed in giggles on the bed.

In the middle of this laughing fest, Charlotte woke up. I was laughing so hard my stomach hurt. Poor Charlotte looked up at me totally confused. Whatever reactions she might have been expecting from me at this point, uncontrollable laughing would not have been one of them. To say I felt guilty is woefully inadequate. My daughter woke up from such a devastating operation to find her mother laughing so hard she could barely breathe.

Gaining control of myself, I managed to explain what I was laughing at and, eventually, Charlotte thought it funny too. We didn't even mention her arm.

In retrospect, it was the best possible thing that could have happened. Laughter prevented my heart from breaking on that day. It lifted my spirits and made me feel that whilst we can still laugh, we will survive. I was able to approach our situation with renewed

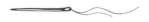

confidence. And Charlotte seeing me laughing made her feel that surely, everything was going to be okay. She saw my reaction and followed suit.

There were many times with Charlotte, my mum and Pat when even during the darkest of times we would find something to laugh at.

Pat and I went together for her test results to tell us if she had breast cancer. We particularly dreaded the news because this would be the third time she had suffered from cancer and chemotherapy would not be available to her as a treatment.

I hadn't met this particular consultant before and Pat described him as being intimidating at a first meeting. 'Well,' I told her, 'he won't intimidate me.' We sat in the consulting room awaiting his arrival. Startling us, the door flew open and in burst a rather large, dishevelled looking man carrying an armful of files. Flinging his files down loudly on the desk and pointing at my sister he barked, 'Uncross your legs please.' In perfect synchronization, Pat and I sat bolt upright and uncrossed our legs. Totally intimidated, I felt like a child back at school. My sister has a way of reducing me to laughter by a sideways glance. I could feel what we called 'giggle mode' coming on so I didn't dare look at her.

The consultant, Mr Jeffries, went to raise my sister's arm to examine her. A strong electrical charge crackled between them. The charge was so strong that Mr Jeffries stumbled back in surprise and lost his footing. But for the bed behind him, he would have been flat on his backside on the floor. In his shock he blurted out, 'What the f…,' but quickly recovered, just in the nick of time. Somehow Pat and I managed to control ourselves until we were back in the hospital corridor. She met my eye and we crumpled, bent double with laughter.

Mr Jeffries had just told Pat that her tests were positive for late stage breast cancer.

The gift of our, sometimes, strange sense of humour came from Mum. The night before she passed away, I spent all night lay beside her on her bed. We spent the whole time giggling like children about the most bizarre things. Mum was hallucinating but she knew it. On a tray at the side of her bed was a glass and a bottle of water. She pointed to it and whispered to me, 'There's a little man sitting on the tray.'

I thought I should follow along so I asked, 'What is he doing?'

'What is who doing?' she asked.

'The little man.'

'What little man? There is no little man.' she said. 'I'm the one taking all the drugs. If you can see a little man, there must be something wrong with you.'

She laughed and said, 'Will you stop making me laugh so much, I am supposed to be ill.' It was a wonderful night. I will remember it forever.

Humour serves me as a coping mechanism though not by way of denying the truth of a situation. Instead it reframes reality for me and softens the blow. It will help you too.

THE BEST MEDICINE

Studies show that laughter boosts the immune system and decreases stress hormones. Given that stress has a role in illnesses such as headaches, anxiety disorders, depression, heart disease, and, possibly, even cancer, it makes sense to laugh more. Chemicals are produced when we laugh that act as natural painkillers and the physical process of laughing positively stimulates all the physiological systems of the body.

Life in all of its forms can be ridiculous; laugh at it. Look for the funny side. Watch funny movies, maybe join a laughter club. Laughter clubs were founded by Dr. Madan Kataria in Mumbai, India in 1995. Since that time the laughter movement has grown, with clubs now in over sixty-five countries including the UK and USA. I think it's telling that many of these clubs take place in the workplace. People who laugh together are more productive together.

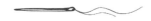

THE T IN CONCEPT IS FOR TRYING NEW THINGS

This means learning new things and having new experiences.

'As long as you're green, you're growing. As soon as you're ripe you start to rot.'

I love this quotation by Ray Kroc, the American businessman behind the success of the food chain McDonalds.

Calling a person *green* is sometimes meant in a derogatory way. It means they are inexperienced or naïve. A green person is one who is new to something and doesn't know much. Unless you have never moved off the spot since the day you were born, you will remember feeling *green* at some point in your life. We all do.

Whatever you do in life, you have to start at the beginning when, chances are, you know little or nothing at all. Feeling green for some people means feeling uncomfortable. As a young person, I hated the first few days of a new job. I felt green and it made me uncomfortable. It was my lack of confidence and the fear of looking foolish. Maturity and experience helped me to overcome that particular fear, but it took a while.

At university, it pained me to see young, bright and intelligent students hold themselves back because of fears such as this. Another 'off curriculum' class. Like me, some of these students will outgrow their fear, but others won't. Some people never overcome the fear of making a fool of themselves. It is crippling because it prevents them from doing something new.

Further education sometimes comes up in conversation when I'm coaching. I might suggest a class or course of some kind. So many times I hear, 'Oh no. I was hopeless at school. I would make a complete fool of myself.' This has to be tackled because new learning and experiencing new things is essential to well-being and life satisfaction.

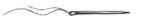

I am an avid supporter of lifelong learning and Kroc's quotation reminds me how important it really is.

GREEN IS GOOD

The point is, green is good. Green is more than good. Let me convince you.

Green means you are at the beginning stages and about to learn something new. The new research linking learning with well-being and satisfaction is overwhelming. Until recently, the benefits of learning have mostly been associated with employability and the economy. In today's economic climate, this is more important than ever. Learning is related to increased earnings and employability and, of course, that indirectly links to well-being.

However, I am more interested in the research that supports my own experience. New learning has direct benefits to personal happiness and well-being levels across the age span.

BACK TO SCHOOL

Soon after Robin and I had created our 'new life' plan, I decided to take an interior design course. Clients of our business often sought my advice on interiors and I felt it would be an idea to do some formal training. An additional benefit would be that Robin and I would spend our working days apart for a while. We were still living with Sword of Damocles. At any time we might discover or hear something that would send us hurtling back into The Twilight Zone. Working together meant we struggled to forget about it even for a short while. We couldn't look at each other without being reminded that anytime now the world could come crashing down. So I started the course.

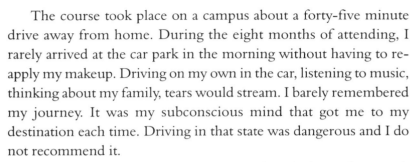

The course took place on a campus about a forty-five minute drive away from home. During the eight months of attending, I rarely arrived at the car park in the morning without having to re-apply my makeup. Driving on my own in the car, listening to music, thinking about my family, tears would stream. I barely remembered my journey. It was my subconscious mind that got me to my destination each time. Driving in that state was dangerous and I do not recommend it.

A major part of the course was practical, including colour work and technical drawing. Additionally, there was a class of decorative painting techniques, which was very fashionable at the time. I was completely green in this class. I had never considered myself to be creative in that way. Nevertheless, I was excited about it. The thing about taking a class is that everyone else there is in the same position. The process of learning about and experimenting with paint brought out creativity I never dreamed I had. I spent hours in the 'zone' or experiencing what positive psychologist, Mihaly Csikszentmihalyi calls 'flow.'

Flow refers to the psychology of the optimal experience. Have you ever been doing something and been concentrating so much that you lost track of time? It's an experience where you almost become unaware of yourself. For example, you forget your aches and pains and you even forget to eat. You are so focused on what you are doing that you become totally unaware of what's going on around you. That's the feeling of flow. Being in flow allows you to forget all of your problems and that's what it did for me. Once the activity was over, in this instance it was painting, I felt rested, relaxed and satisfied – no matter how good or bad the final product of my efforts.

My journey home from class was so different from the journey there. I felt more positive and far more confident about dealing with life's challenges.

Coincidentally, (except that I don't believe in coincidences) one

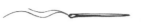

of the subjects covered on the course was Art History and I loved it. Later I went on to do a part-time degree in Art and Design History.

What does all this have to do with happiness and well-being? Well, learning broadens horizons. It opens doors that lead to other enjoyable beneficial experiences. This we know. For example, my degree allowed me to go on to volunteer at the art gallery, which gave me the confidence to consider lecturing, which, ultimately, led me to writing and coaching. The overwhelming research I mentioned previously has shown that new learning inspires confidence and helps to develop capabilities and resources. It encourages social interaction and gives a sense of belonging. Everyone is in the 'same boat' and therefore immediately has something in common. Learning gives purpose and meaning to life. It promotes optimism and increases resilience. Learning at any age helps people feel more able to deal with problems and anxieties.

If that hasn't convinced you to become a lifelong learner maybe this will:

You will, no doubt, have heard the saying, 'You can't teach an old dog new tricks.' This was believed because, up until the last thirty years or so, scientists had thought the brain completed its development when we reached our mid-thirties. We now know better. More recent research has demonstrated that our brain continues to grow and change. The brain achieves this by continuing to rewire and create new neural circuits at any age. This capability is called 'neuroplasticity' and is kicked into action by new learning and experiences. The more new learning you do, the more connections are made in your brain. Many of these connections may be redundant but still add to the richness or plasticity of the brain. If, for any reason, some connections are lost, it means you have more in reserve. The more new learning or education you have, the less likely you are to experience the loss of mental functions or cognitive decline. Cognitive decline is a key feature of dementia.

A collaborative study carried out by scientists from universities

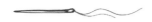

in Cambridge, Sheffield, Newcastle and Finland found that where people with more education might have showed biological signs of dementia at death, they were less likely to have displayed the symptoms of it while they were alive.

To my knowledge, there doesn't seem to be evidence that learning prevents the onset of dementia, but it does appear to delay the appearance of its symptoms.

When Kroc gave us the quotation about being green, he didn't have the science to support him. We have it now and it cannot be ignored.

What to do about it? The answer is easy and fun. Be curious, go back to being a beginner, go back to being green. A new experience can be as easy as taking a different route to work in the morning. It doesn't have to mean embarking on a huge adventure, although that would be good. Neither do you have to commit to full-time learning or taking a degree to learn something new. Read a book on a subject you wouldn't normally be interested in. Learn to dance or flower arrange. Take up painting or learn a language, perhaps take a computer class. I don't need to tell you: the list is endless. Once you have mastered something, try something else.

A tip to make the most of your new learning and new experience is to combine them. You do this when you read about how to do something and go on to put it into practice. Combining the two strengthens the connections made in your brain and helps you to store what you learn into long-term memory. Making longer lasting synaptic connections (the process by which a neuron passes a signal to another cell) takes focused concentration. The kind of attention found in Csikszentmihalyi's flow experience.

CREATING FLOW

Choose something you think you will enjoy doing. Obviously, this

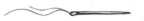

will be different for everyone. However, the criteria that help to cultivate the experience are the same:

a) Strike the right balance between the challenge the activity presents to you and your skill level. The challenge must not be so difficult that you feel unable to do it, or so easy you will soon become bored.
b) Break the activity down into chunks. Have definite goals and know what you want to achieve for each step.
c) Choose an activity that gives instant feedback on your performance. So, for instance, when I was painting, I could see with each stroke if I was achieving the desired effect.

Thanks to new sciences, we are understanding more and more about how our brains work. It's up to you to put the findings of research into practice to help you in your own life.

In the short term, trying something new helped me through a dreadful time in my life. Call it escapism, if you will. It allowed me to escape from my all-encompassing problems by giving me something else to focus on. When I returned to my problems, I was stronger. I had a much clearer and more effective mind. Long term, it opened doors that led me to a much more fulfilling and satisfying life.

There is no doubt that trying new things increases happiness and well-being levels. Just commit to being *green*, and learn to enjoy it.

Remember the words of the American basketball player, John Wooden. 'It's what you learn after you know it all that counts.'

KICK-START WITH THE CONCEPT

That's the Conroy Concept of Well-being. The ideas are presented

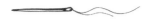
under seven subject headings, but it's clear to see that they are interconnected. For example, the better your relationships, the more pleasure and fun you are likely to have, and the other way around. The more you learn about things, such as health, the more likely you are to want to exercise. Living more in the present helps with the experience of flow, which produces deeper learning and so on.

One of the things I like about the Concept is that you can start to do something immediately, and it doesn't have to cost a penny – only your attention and a little bit of effort. Let the Conroy Concept kick-start you to happiness.

CHAPTER FIVE

LET IT GO AND GIVE THANKS:
FORGIVENESS AND APPRECIATION

Two things underpinning the Conroy Concept of Happiness and Well-being are Forgiveness and Appreciation. Without mastering these two things, your life will be lacking.

FORGIVE AND FORGET?

Forgiveness is a principle of most of the world's religions. God forgives us and we should forgive each other. We have tremendous admiration for people like Gandhi and Nelson Mandela who were capable of such amazing acts of forgiveness. Some people are even able to forgive their children's killers and we gasp in awe when we hear such stories. In general, we accept that forgiveness is a moral and right thing to do.

Psychological studies are now telling us that it's also a healthy thing to do. Being able to forgive is crucial to happiness and well-being. It helps us to move forward with a clean slate and hope for the future. Forgiveness is empowering and increases our self-esteem. It decreases levels of depression, anxiety and anger, and, therefore, the likelihood of heart disease. I believe this wholeheartedly, but I also believe it is an incredibly challenging

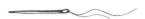

thing to do. Throughout my life there have been times where I found the ability to forgive challenging, to say the least. However, through research and experience, I have discovered some simple but effective tools to help with the process. I am going to share them with you. Before I do that, let me first explain what I mean by forgiveness.

At some time or another in your life, you will have been hurt by other people. You might be hurting now. Somebody has done something or said something to offend you. It happens to all of us. We have disagreements, perhaps with colleagues or friends, and for a while feel affronted. Thinking rationally, most of us can agree with the statement, 'There are three sides to every argument: your side, the other side, and the right side.' Time heals and we do come to understand that there could have been fault on both sides. Once we have accepted that, it's easier to move on.

What about the other hurts? Those often caused by people we care about the most? Disagreements with people we care about can be the fiercest and most damaging. We are more emotionally involved. There is more at stake and more to lose. Unfortunately, when emotions are involved, rational thinking flies through the window. Every now and then something happens and understanding or healing seems to be impossible. We are wounded and it leaves a lasting feeling of bitterness and resentment. And, yes, I am talking from experience.

BITTERNESS AND RESENTMENT

I mentioned that, as a teenager, the relationship with my mother was turbulent. One day, after having had a particularly nasty argument the night before, I came home from work to find all my clothes and belongings piled neatly on my bed. No words necessary. It was my marching orders. I was deeply hurt and panicking

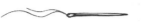

because I had nowhere to go. A mixture of anger, fear and hurt seared through my stomach like red hot coals. I shakily gathered my things and left.

It was eight years before I saw Mum again. During that time I married and gave birth to my first child. I felt intensely wounded. I was bitter and resentful about the fight, the way I left, and the fact that my mother was absent for two of the most momentous occasions in my life.

Each time I thought about what happened, even years later, it was as clear in my mind as if it had happened the day before. It felt like I was re-living the whole thing again and I still felt the hot coals searing through my stomach. That feeling was every bit as powerful and crippling as it had been on the day of the incident. As much as I tried to suppress the feeling, it just wouldn't go away. And, although I feigned indifference, I really missed my mum. I realized there was only one thing to do. To quote John Ruskin, 'It is better to lose your pride with someone you love rather than lose that someone you love with your useless pride.'

One morning after a trip to the park with my baby boy, I went to my mother's house and knocked on the door. I didn't even know what I was going to say.

It took a few seconds for her to recognize me with babe in arms, and then her face crumpled. She wrapped us in her arms and wept.

I am ashamed to say it but that was the first time I had even considered my mother's suffering.

We didn't discuss or thrash out our differences, and our relationship was never the same. Instead, we developed a new relationship, one that included mutual respect and, eventually, we became friends. As I said, we didn't finally resolve these early issues until the end of her life. By which time the searing hot coals had long since burnt themselves out.

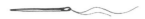

THE MIND-BODY CONNECTION

In recent years, we have come to understand exactly how powerful the mind-body connection is – the idea that your body responds to your emotions. Equally, we know that your emotions respond to your thoughts. A simple way to demonstrate how this plays out is to think about when you have a negative thought, such as 'I am going to lose my job.' That leads to negative emotions like stress and worry, which in turn leads to negative physiology, for example stomach ulcers, headaches, and even high blood pressure or heart disease.

You could think of it this way: every thought you have produces a chemical in your body. Positive thoughts produce positive chemicals; negative thoughts produce negative chemicals.

Each time I thought about the fight I had with Mum, which was often, I felt the bitterness and resentment all over again. The chemicals released into my body were so toxic I felt a physical, searing pain in my stomach. Instinctively, I knew I had to let it go or I was going to be ill, and there's the rub. *I* was going to be ill, not Mum. My resentment was harming only me. 'Unforgiveness is like drinking poison and expecting the other person to die' (*author unknown*). I let go of the resentment and anger towards my mother. I didn't feel any need to hurt back. I accepted the situation and we moved on.

WHAT IS FORGIVENESS?

Mum and I moved on from the past into a different relationship. Does that mean we forgave each other? Some religions believe that repentance is necessary before true forgiveness can take place. Neither Mum nor I apologized or even admitted responsibility for the part

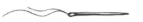

each of us played. There was a kind of knowing; a silent agreement that remained unspoken between us. For our relationship, that was enough. I suppose it's up to you what you are prepared to accept.

I believe I forgave. The resentment and bitterness I felt towards Mum was released from me almost the moment I knocked on her door. Later, when I thought about her, I felt a calm peacefulness that signified to me that, on my part, forgiveness had taken place.

The 'forget' part, I find tricky. How can you forget an experience that is burned into your memory? You can't 'unknow' or 'unexperience'. I actually don't think you should forget the experience. In fact, I think quite the opposite. You need to remember hurtful experiences so that you can learn from them. Just as you would hope to learn from any other negative experiences. If you don't learn, you are in danger of putting yourself back in the same position and being hurt again.

What surely needs to be forgotten is the anger, bitterness and resentment surrounding the experience.

Although it is easier to be hurt by those we love, it is easier to forgive them too. I confess, I have found it more challenging to forgive wrongdoing in other relationships. Some people are easier to forgive than others. Sometimes it is easier to forgive when the other person is sorry. Each incident with each person needs to be considered differently.

The point is, you are going to be hurt – possibly many times by many different people in your life. It's what you choose to do about it that is important. Stay stuck with the anger, bitterness and resentment and let the past rule your future? Or take a first step towards health and well-being and decide to forgive.

Don't Deny your Feelings

Forgiveness does not mean you condone the bad behaviour or that you are letting the offender 'get away with it'. Neither do you have to reconcile with the offender or even see them again if you don't want to. Forgiveness does not mean you are denying your feelings. There is a time for anger, sadness and hurt, and a time to let it go.

Of all the things I am suggesting you do throughout this book, forgiving someone who has hurt you is probably the most difficult thing of all. However, carrying around anger and resentment about something, especially something from years ago, gets in the way of your happiness and well-being. It is also a sure-fire way to illness and even early death. If for the benefit of no-one else, forgive for yourself.

EXERCISE 9:
SEVEN STEPS TO HELP BUILD YOUR FORGIVENESS MUSCLE

As with any new behaviour or skill, forgiveness takes practise so you need to start with something small. Think of something somebody did to you that might have irritated you just a little bit. Perhaps something a colleague said to you that you didn't like. Use that example to implement the following process. Build your forgiveness muscle. That way it will come easier to you when you really need it.

You will need pen and paper and somewhere to sit quietly and undisturbed for about thirty minutes.

1) Make the decision to *intend* to forgive.
2) Get clear about the issue by writing down exactly what happened.
3) Put a name to your feelings. If you were angry, try to uncover the feelings beneath the anger. Were you disappointed? Did you feel rejected or abandoned? Humiliated or abused? Deceived or cheated? Be honest with yourself about this. Sometimes the act of naming your true feelings alone can release anger and lessen the depth of feeling.
4) Close your eyes and take a few long deep breaths. Be aware of the

inhale and the exhale. Imagine all the feelings you have written down on your paper coming together in the form of a ball of thick black smoke. Feel this 'bad feeling' smoke circulating around your body. Take a deep breath in, letting your tummy rise as you do so. When you breathe out, imagine blowing the black smoke out through your mouth and out of your body.

Breathe in fresh cleansing breath. Breathe out thick black smoke. Continue visualizing the black smoke emptying out of your body with every exhale until it has all gone. When your body feels cleansed, take a long deep breath in and out – feel yourself relax. Open your eyes. This is known as the black smoke meditation.

5) Ask yourself the following questions and write down your answers. If you were to do to someone else what this person did to you, what might your reason be for behaving that way? Can you think of different reasons?

Now remember a time when you hurt someone and they forgave you. (We are all capable of hurting others. There must be at least one time?) How did it feel to be forgiven? Did you feel relieved? At peace? Were you thankful?

6) The following is an adaptation of a Buddhist meditation, known as the Loving Kindness meditation, intended to sweeten and change negative patterns of the mind. It serves our purpose perfectly. Sit in a comfortable position and close your eyes. Take a few long, deep breaths and feel your body relax. Think of someone you love deeply – a partner, a child, a parent, or even a pet. Let the feeling of love flow. For me, there is nothing like the sound of giggling babies or seeing a cute puppy to evoke this feeling. Anything that gives you that lovely warm glow will do. When you feel that lovely feeling, say to yourself, 'Let me be filled with loving kindness and let me be at peace.'

Hold the feeling and now imagine your family and friends. Extend the feeling to them and silently repeat, 'May you be filled with loving kindness and be at peace.' Keep thinking back to the original source of warmth to strengthen the feeling. Now think of the person who

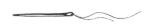

hurt you. Try to hold the feeling and, whilst thinking of them, repeat, 'May you be filled with loving kindness and be at peace.' End the process by thinking back to the original source to strengthen your feeling and once again say to yourself, 'May *I* be filled with loving kindness and be at peace.' Take a few long, deep breaths and end the meditation.

Don't be concerned if you lose the warmth when you think of the wrongdoer or if other feelings come up. Let them come up, let them go. Carry on with the meditation and relax. You can try again and it will get easier each time.

7) Letter of forgiveness.

Finally, I want you to write to the person who hurt you and tell them you forgive them. Write without blame if you can but state how their actions made you feel. Tell them you forgive them or tell them of your intentions to forgive, and wish them well... then tear up the letter or burn it – ceremoniously.

Forgiveness takes effort. Being willing to forgive is the first step. Keep repeating the seven steps until you can think about the incident and the person who hurt you differently. When you do, you will be able to move on with a clean slate. Now you are no longer a victim. Now, instead of ruminating and worrying about what happened to you, you can remember that you forgave. You took control and changed the way you feel. Now, you can be at peace and you are increasing your levels of happiness and well-being.

LEARN A LIFE LESSON FROM THE ERASER PENCIL

It has a short life, yet it can make a significant mark – just like you.
It is not a pen.
Its mistakes can be corrected with effort, but it often means standing the pencil on its head.
Instead of the power that the world advocates, seek love.

Instead of revenge, seek to forgive.
For the pencil, like you, what is inside, not outside, is responsible for its mark.
The pencil needs to be ground down and sharpened regularly, so don't despise the sharpening that you must undergo.
Often the hurts and wounds you feel as painful can be your own sharpening.
(Worthington, 2006)

APPRECIATION

When you were a child did your parents ever say, 'You should count your blessings?' Mine did. Whenever I complained about anything, Mum would admonish me by saying, 'You need to count your blessings young lady. You have no right to complain. You should be grateful for what you have.' Consequently, being grateful has always had a sermonizing ring to it for me. The word 'grateful' itself conjures up feelings of shame and obligation. Although it means pretty much the same thing, I prefer to use the word 'appreciation'.

'Understanding of the full worth of something; recognition and enjoyment of the good qualities of someone or something, or showing pleasure for something somebody does for you.'

That's what appreciation means. Important to us because, like forgiveness, appreciation is receiving much scientific attention right now. Studies are showing that an appreciative nature plays a significant role in increasing happiness and well-being. It isn't only about lifting your mood at the time, although it will do that. Making a conscious effort to be more appreciative improves physical health, improves relationships, and increases your general satisfaction with life. Appreciation will help you through the most testing of times.

Over the years many people have asked me the question, 'Do

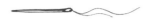

you ever wonder, why you?' The honest answer to that is, 'Never.' I admit to occasionally feeling sorry for myself, but never for long.

FROM THE MOUTHS OF BABES

When it was discovered that Charlotte had cancer, we were sent for further investigations to a hospital in Birmingham, which is about a two and a half hour drive from where we lived. We arrived at what had been described to us as a Victorian garden hospital. It may well once have been as pleasant as that sounds. In fact, it turned out to be a dilapidated, gloomy building that had been added to over the years. The original architect's design had suffered from its own numerous, cancerous growths. The building itself looked undernourished and diseased. Apparently, its original raison d'être was to encourage wellness and recuperation; it had the opposite effect on us. I didn't even want to go inside.

While Robin filled in the necessary paperwork, Charlotte and I went up to the ward. We walked through the doors and I stopped dead in my tracks. The beds lining the ward were occupied by children of all ages. Some of them were hooked up to drips, some had limbs missing, all of them had the unmistakable pallor that says *'seriously ill'* and most of them were without hair. I had never seen anything like it in my life. It felt like we'd walked into a war zone. I started to shake and was rooted to the spot. My first coherent thought was, 'We are not staying here.' Suddenly, I felt a tiny, warm hand slip into mine. Shaking my hand for attention, Charlotte looked up at me and said:

'Never mind, Mummy – we'll probably get used to it tomorrow.'

So far on this horrible journey, most of my thoughts had been totally selfish. 'What was I going to do? How would I cope with Charlotte's illness? How could I bear to stay in this hospital?' I was thinking only about myself, as if I were a victim. Jolted out of my selfish reverie, I sank to my knees and, with my heart bursting, I thanked God

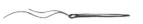

for my daughter. I held her tight and told her I loved her. Here was this gorgeous little girl, who must have been so confused and frightened herself, comforting me. Down there on my knees I began to feel a strong sense of determination surging through me. Finally, I rose to my feet and, taking Charlotte's hand, I said, 'Right, that's it. Come on. We are going to do this and *you*… are going to get better.'

I had so much to appreciate. My daughter's inspirational strength and courage, my lovely husband, my boys, the medical staff who treated us with such warmth and compassion, the doctors who went way beyond the call of duty to help us, and the friends and family who did rally round. The list was endless.

It really is true that it's not what happens to you but how you choose to deal with it that counts, and make no mistake, you do have a choice.

It was during our stay at Birmingham that we discovered Charlotte had an underlying condition that predisposed her to cancer in the first place. It was here that the doctors realized that treatment with chemotherapy was too dangerous to be an option. The only 'treatment' option was to amputate. Of course, we were horror struck. However, it wasn't too long before we were writing a letter of appreciation to Charlotte's surgeon for saving her life.

The quantum physicist, Max Planck, said, 'If you change the way you look at things, the things you look at change.'

Charlotte understood, even at such a young age, that what happened to her could have been so much worse. Her time spent in children's cancer wards taught all of us that.

ALWAYS SOMETHING TO APPRECIATE

Pat had cancer four times, with all the anguish, pain and hurt that it entails. She had operations that went wrong, she lost her hair – twice – and had heart problems caused by the supposed cures, she

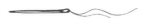

couldn't have children – the list goes on. The full account of what happened to her reads like a horror story. If anyone is entitled to ask 'Why me?', it's her. I have never once heard her ask that question, either. Whenever she is in hospital, she can always be found chatting with someone who has no visitors. She always manages to find someone who, in some way, is in a worse position than herself to talk to and try to lift their spirits. 'I'm so glad I have family,' is something she often says.

Incidentally, you need never suffer alone if you or a family member has cancer. A group who deserve a special mention here in terms of our appreciation is the Macmillan cancer support organization. Called upon by us for all three Conroy women – the angels who are the Macmillan nurses were there for us with advice, physical and psychological support. I think a similar organization in the United States is the Cancer Support Community. Either way, these organizations exist to help you. Do not hesitate to give them a call.

I am aware that what happened to my Conroy Women is extreme. I tell their stories to illustrate the point that no matter how dire your situation, there is always something to be thankful for. Pardon the pun here but, thankfully, we don't all have to face such extreme circumstances.

During the course of any given day, negative things happen. The trick is to refuse to give them power. On any given day, good things happen too and these are where your focus needs to be. You choose where to place your attention. Get into the habit now of looking for the positive and it will serve you well whenever you meet greater challenges.

Here's an exercise to keep your attention on the positive. It's a positive psychology intervention but its origins go right back with my mother and your mother and probably their mothers too. It's called the gratitude exercise and is based on the idea of counting your blessings.

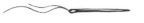

EXERCISE 10:

THE GRATITUDE EXERCISE

Each night before you go to sleep, think about three things you can be thankful for that happened during the day. Some people like to write them down in a journal; it's your choice. They don't have to be big things.

One day, in a hurry to get to work, I had been stuck in what felt like a week-long traffic jam. In my frustration, I was drumming my fingers on the steering wheel and becoming more and more impatient. I looked up and a truck driver beamed a huge smile at me. I smiled back and immediately relaxed. It reminded me to breathe and be present in the moment. He made my morning and it went into my journal that night.

If you struggle with the word 'grateful' too, just ask yourself, 'What went right for me today?' Focus on the positive things that happened.

One of my clients prefers to do this in the mornings about the previous day. She says it puts her in the right frame of mind to start her day. That's the magic of this ever-so-simple technique – it changes your mind-set. You will even find yourself looking for things during the day to think about or write down that night.

When you have been doing this for a while, change the format and only write twice a week. This keeps the exercise fresh and prevents it from becoming a chore.

EXERCISE 11:

APPRECIATION LETTER

I mentioned sending a letter of appreciation to my daughter's surgeon. Try sending a letter of appreciation or a card to someone who has helped you, even in a small way. Imagine how your postman or other

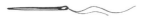

service provider would feel if they received a little card expressing appreciation for what they do.

The fact is, in today's busy world, we often forget the small niceties and it can be those very things that make all the difference, both to the recipient and to you. 'Hem your blessings with thankfulness so they don't unravel.' *(Author unknown.)*

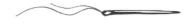

CHAPTER SIX

DON'T DESERVE IT. CAN'T DO IT:
SELF ESTEEM AND CONFIDENCE

Acceptance of the ideas presented in this book is important for increasing your happiness and well-being levels. However, most crucially, you need to accept that you are deserving of happiness in the first place. You can follow the ideas presented here until the cows come home but if you feel underserving of happiness, consciously or otherwise, they will not work for you long-term.

For that reason, I want to talk about your levels of self-esteem and confidence. Healthy levels of self-esteem and confidence are essential to your happiness and to your ability to recover when disaster strikes in your life.

NEW THINKING ABOUT SELF ESTEEM

The only thing to be agreed upon about the subject of self-esteem is that there is a strong correlation between it and your happiness. Apart from that, there seems to be disagreement amongst psychologists about what it is, what causes it, and what can be done about it. Particularly in the United States, there is strong debate about its causes, merits and consequences. For decades, we have been led to believe that low self-esteem is a risk factor for practically all of society's ills. From delinquency to extreme violence and sexual abuse, low self-esteem was thought to be a cause. More and more recent research reveals that there is no hard evidence for this thinking. The 'self-esteem movement' itself, which originated in America in the 1970s to enhance the self-esteem of American citizens, has come under heavy criticism. Some psychologists now believe that attempts to raise self-esteem through specific programmes in schools and churches, actually damaged the young people of America, ultimately producing a generation of narcissistic, young adults. It seems that praising children no matter what and leading them to believe they are brilliant and special has backfired. Instead, it is thought that such practices have encouraged selfishness and a tendency toward overblown views of talent and a craving for attention.

I had to smile, a little ironically, when looking at this research. I was going through the grammar school system in England during the 1970s. I don't think my school or my parents had even heard of the self-esteem movement. I once rushed home from school having attained second place out of thirty-eight in a particularly difficult maths exam and, excitedly, told my father of my achievement. He very crushingly responded by asking why I hadn't come first. At school, which I saw as a place of freedom from my very strict and suffocating home life, I admit to being a tad unruly at times. Possibly, more-so in my physics class because I didn't enjoy the subject. As either retribution or for his own amusement, my physics teacher devised a way to humiliate me that I have never forgotten. At the beginning of each of his sessions, he would make me stand in front of the whole class and he would say, 'You are an imbecile, Christine. What are you?' And, of course, I had to reply, 'I am an imbecile, Sir.' That happened at each class for a full term. I can promise you, I didn't leave my school with overblown views about my talents. I have since recounted this tale to various groups of my students and their response is always the same – they laugh. I laugh too. It is so

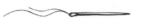

outrageous that it's funny. Of course, it wasn't funny at all. I would hope that somebody dishing out such bullying today would be dismissed from teaching.

WHAT IS SELF-ESTEEM?

There is so much information out there about self-esteem and, as I said, much of it contradictory. I can only answer the question by telling you what I mean by it in the context of how it affects your happiness levels. Put very simply:

Self-esteem is your own opinion of yourself. How you see yourself, and how much you like what you see. It is an emotional feeling about your own self-worth, your worthiness of love, and your worthiness of happiness.

Self-confidence is inextricably linked to your self-esteem and is the judgement you make about your ability to exist in the world. It is your belief in what you can do.

Someone with self-esteem sees themselves as being capable, valued and respected. Approaching life in a positive way, they take responsibility for themselves and their actions and demonstrate respect and care for others. They don't concern themselves too much about what others think of them, but they are open to constructive criticism. People with self-esteem are less judgemental of themselves and of others. Whilst they are prepared to try new things and stretch themselves, they have realistic attitudes towards their capabilities, and are prepared to ask for help when they need it. They like themselves and feel deserving of both love and happiness. You can see how someone who feels like this would also have strong beliefs in their abilities to meet with life's challenges

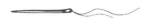

and to reach their life goals, e.g. self-confidence. You will also understand that feeling so good about themselves increases their happiness levels.

There is an argument that says that you either have self-esteem or you don't. My experience doesn't bear this out. I have met people with varying degrees of it, and so describing the opposite of someone with self-esteem I use the terms 'low self-esteem' and 'unhealthy self-esteem'. Those people with unhealthy self-esteem have been badly damaged in some way. They don't merely dislike themselves, they hate themselves to such a degree that they are temporarily or permanently incapable of participating effectively in the world. I include here, for example, those who self-harm and those with severe eating disorders of some kind. People such as these need lots of encouragement and support to help them, either through one-to-one professional therapy, group counselling, or sometimes hospitalization.

On the other hand, I believe that, if we care to admit it, many of us suffer at some point, in some areas of life, from low self–esteem, and I know that practising the Conroy Concept helps.

LOW SELF-ESTEEM

A person with low self-esteem suffers from self-doubt. They often feel inadequate, unworthy, unlovable and fearful. They are judgemental and critical about themselves and can be so about others. Often they are shy, though not always. You can understand how someone who feels this way probably has less belief in their abilities to meet with life's challenges or to reach their life goals. Therefore, you could be forgiven for thinking that people with low self-esteem must be introverted underachievers. You would be wrong. Sometimes it is the highest achievers, striving to prove to themselves and to others that they are worthy, who suffer the most from low self-esteem. Or, the perfectionist who isn't that way because their standards are high, but because they are at pains to avoid being seen as failures. Some people refuse to admit having low self-esteem to themselves, let alone to others. Denial causes its own problems. Low self-esteem is complicated and certainly difficult to understand. It is, however, worth the effort to understand.

Low self-esteem may or may not be a contributory factor to delinquency and violence. However, there is no doubt that having these feelings, at any level, leads to self-defeating beliefs and behaviours that, if they don't ruin your life, will very definitely sabotage your happiness. And this is where my interest lies.

EXERCISE 12: (IN THREE PARTS)
DO YOU HAVE PROBLEMS WITH SECS? PART ONE.

SECS is an abbreviation I use to mean suffering from either low Self-Esteem, lack of Confidence, Shyness, or all three. Take a pen and paper, a cup of tea or coffee, and give yourself some time. Answer the following questions. Answer the first part of each question quickly writing the very first answer that comes to you. Take a little more time over the second part of the question but don't censor yourself, say whatever comes into your mind. In general:

1) Do you suffer from low Self-Esteem? Yes or No.
   If so, how do you think it affects you?
2) Do you suffer from lack of Confidence? Yes or No.
   If so, how do you think it affects you?
3) Do you suffer from Shyness? Yes or No.
   If so, how do you think it affects you?

If you were unable to answer a definitive yes or no to the first part of those questions, don't worry. Many people answer 'sometimes'

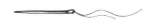

or 'it depends on the situation'. My aim here is not diagnosis, but to get you to think about it. There are self-esteem scales that you can take online that will help you if you feel you need it. I think you will have a good idea yourself.

If you are already aware that you have one or all of these, there are some things you need to know. First of all, if you suffer from SECS or any part thereof, you are like millions of others. Secondly, it is not your fault, and thirdly, it is nothing to be ashamed of. However, once you know there is an issue, what you do about it is your choice. It may not feel like it right now, but you are in control. You can do something about it.

I believe the key to positive change is self-knowledge. Becoming aware of your beliefs and understanding your behaviour.

EXERCISE 12:
PART TWO

Go back to your answer to the second part of question one. Ask yourself why you think you behave that way.

Let me give you an example using Mary.

Mary answered question one above with a definite yes. She was aware of her low self-esteem. Answering the second part she told me about her job. She didn't much like her current position in administration where she worked for her company part-time. She rather liked the idea of working in the sales department. When a position in sales became available, her boss said she should apply. Mary's immediate thought to herself was, 'Oh no, I can't possibly do that.' Although she was initially pleased that her boss thought she could do it, she later decided he was just being nice. In reality, she felt he knew she wouldn't even get an interview. Right up until

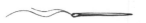

the closing date, she thought about putting in her application. In the end, she decided she was probably better staying where she was, doing what she knew. She is still in administration.

I asked her why she thought she behaved in such a way. Unfortunately, her answer was one that I hear all the time. She told me that, deep down, she felt she wasn't good enough. She also felt that by applying and failing to get the job, she would make a fool of herself in front of everyone.

What was your answer?

Mary thought she couldn't (self-defeating thought) apply for the job because she knew she wasn't good enough (self-defeating belief). So she let the opportunity go (self-defeating behaviour). She wanted the job but sabotaged the possibility of getting it by not applying in the first place. Now answer the second part of questions two and three in Part One above.

EXERCISE 12:
PART THREE

The next step in the exercise involves having the courage to do a little bit of delving into that deep dark place we often blame for all of our faults – the past. But only for a little while, and not for any 're-living of the moment' catharsis. Just to think about the experiences you have had, either in your childhood but also since then, that may have planted the seeds for some of your beliefs.

Mary's story is somewhat stereotypical but nonetheless debilitating for her. She was brought up in a very traditional home where her father worked and her mother stayed home to look after her and her older brother. She had good memories of her childhood. Nevertheless, even though her parents were loving towards her, growing up she was always conscious that her brother was the favourite in the house. Whenever her brother achieved anything, their parents always made more fuss of him and seemed more proud than they were of Mary's achievements. Over time, she began to feel her own achievements didn't matter and so she stopped trying.

As an adult, Mary lacked confidence and often experienced self-doubt, but she learned to live with it and life was okay. When she married and had a family, just as her mum before her, she stayed home to look after her children believing this was the key to a happy marriage. Everything was fine until one by one her children left home for college or university. She was miserable. Mary resisted the idea of going out to work because she felt guilty and, anyway, she couldn't think of anything she would be able to do. Eventually, and with her husband's encouragement, she applied for her current part-time position, which meant she would still be able to care for her home and husband. Getting the first job she applied for boosted her confidence and, for a while, she enjoyed the work.

Chatting one lunchtime, Mary told a colleague how surprised she had been when she was offered the job, given that she was so nervous during the interview. The colleague replied, 'Knowing Bill, [the interviewer] you probably only got the job because you were the last one interviewed and the only one he remembered.' 'Ah,' Mary thought to herself, 'so, that's why I got the job.' This confirmed all of Mary's self-doubts. It confirmed to her that she wasn't as good as she thought she was at interviews and that she was only in her current job by default. When the sales position came up, she believed that she was not good enough and would fail at the interview.

These are the facts as Mary saw them.

We talked about her parents' method of parenting, objectively and without criticism, in an attempt to understand why any parent might be more supportive of one child. Apart from loving one child more than the other (Mary said she always felt loved), what other reasons could there be? Now that Mary was openly and rationally

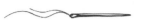

discussing the situation, the answer was obvious to her. Immediately she knew it was that her parents' traditional thinking led them to believe that of the two of them, it was more important for her brother to receive a good education and be successful. He was the one who needed good employment because he would be the one having to work to support his family.

Looking back at this situation as an adult, Mary was able to rationalize her parents' behaviour. As her father had passed away, the next step for Mary, if she felt able, would be to talk to her mother about it in a loving and supportive way. Her self-esteem issues may not miraculously disappear, but understanding was the first step to a new way of thinking for her that could encourage her to at least try for a new position the next time.

A person with low self-esteem tends to focus only on their weaknesses and is quick to believe the negative about him- or herself. In fact, they tend only to see the negative and disregard the positive, just as Mary did when her boss said she should apply for the sales position. Instead of seeing that suggestion as him having faith in her, she thought he was 'just being nice'. When her colleague told her she probably only got the job because she was the only one the interviewer could remember, Mary believed it. Instead she should question the colleague's motives for the comment. What evidence did the colleague have for saying that? How do we know it's true? Why would someone say something like that when Mary was confessing to being a nervous interviewee?

Start to question your own beliefs. Especially if you look back to the past and see a pattern of self-defeating behaviour. Remember beliefs are not facts. Beliefs are simply thoughts you keep thinking and your thoughts are not necessarily true.

Mary can look at her past now and recognize that the foundation of the beliefs causing her pattern of self-defeating behaviour was shaky. That's a good place to start. The next time a position in sales becomes available, I have a strong feeling Mary will apply.

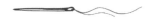

LACK OF SELF-CONFIDENCE

During the first meeting with ninety apprehensive first year students, I always introduced myself and warmly welcomed them to the university. Next, I introduced them to the subject, which in this case was Design History, and told them what to expect from the course. After ten minutes or so, they would begin to relax. Once I had reached the stage where the students were comfortable, I would walk around the lecture theatre and then say, 'I am now going to choose someone to come down to the front and talk to the rest of the group for five minutes or so about what design means to them.' Within a split second, the atmosphere in the room fell like a stone from a high rise building. I could smell the fear. The students would literally curl up in their seats and look anywhere else but at me. I didn't allow them to suffer too long before confessing that I was, in fact, teasing them and had no intention of making anyone stand up and speak. At that point the students would collapse with sheer relief followed by very nervous laughter.

Immediately, I would ask for a raise of hands from anyone who had felt their heart beat faster, their palms get sweaty, their breathing become faster and shallower, possibly feel their stomach knot? Most of their hands would go up and I would ask them why. Somebody always shouted 'fear'.

Fear of what? I asked them to really think about what went through their minds to make them feel so bad. No matter the group or their ages, as mature students were also represented, the answers were always the same. 'I can't talk in front of all these people.' 'She [meaning me] is going to think I'm an idiot.' 'What if my mind goes blank?' 'Everyone will judge me.' 'I look fat and ugly.' 'They will laugh at me.' 'I am going to look stupid.' 'I will make a fool of myself.' 'I will fail.'

The point of this exercise was to alert them to the fact that the single most debilitating thing that stops people from achieving their

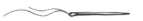

goals and becoming successful is FEAR. Fear of the very same things they were previously afraid of when I suggested I might choose them to speak. In addition, as designers, if they were afraid of being laughed at or being seen as stupid or failing, they would never produce anything original. Designing is all about experiment and trial and error. Getting things wrong. Learning from mistakes and trying again. Of course, this doesn't only apply to designers. The exercise also demonstrates pretty spectacularly that everyone feels the same way. I would refer back to this exercise when I talked to them about personal development because within a matter of seconds it produces a perfect example of *thinging*. If you remember:

Ruminating – churning the same thing over and over

Imagining – what if?

Exaggerating – making something worse than it is

Everyone lacks the confidence to do things they don't know how to do. Practise makes you better at something and, the better you get, the more your confidence grows. Step by step or even small baby steps at first is fine until you feel a little braver and you are ready to take a bigger step.

When I first started public speaking, my nerves were so bad I felt physically sick. Each time, I almost backed out because I didn't think I could do it. Throughout the whole time I was on stage, my stomach was so tense that, by the end, it felt as though I had done a hundred sit ups. I decided to find training to help me build my confidence and joined a speaker's club. Week by week I became better and better. Eventually, even winning a speaking award. Now, I still get nervous but it's more about helping the audience benefit from my message than about how I am going to perform.

I feel passionately about teaching the art of public speaking. Obviously, not everyone wants to stand up and speak to, or entertain, large groups of people. It isn't just about that. If you think about it, all speaking is public speaking. These days if you are going for an interview, it's quite possible to be facing a panel of five or six.

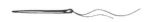

You might need to give presentations or sell something. I would tell my students that if you can stand up in front of more than one person and speak confidently, you are well ahead of your competition in the workplace. Public speaking is something most people feel they would rather die than do.

I feel it necessary here to justify my teasing of the students. At the end of my module with them, when I asked for volunteers to come down and speak to the class, I would find it difficult to choose amongst all the hands that would fly up. It was satisfying for all of us to note their progress.

SHYNESS

Shyness can be a part of low self-esteem and a lack of confidence but it doesn't have to be. You might just be shy. When I talk about shyness in this instance, I am not talking about those who are so acutely shy they are social phobic. Again, those with social phobia are better served by those qualified to help in that particular area. I mean those people whose shyness presents them with difficulties that are not enough to stop them from doing what they want to do, but are often enough to make them, and sometimes those around them, miserable.

Are you anxious in certain social situations, concerned that you don't have anything to say, or that you might say the inappropriate thing? Do you become embarrassed when the attention is focused on you? Are you afraid you might make a negative impression? If the answer is yes to any of those questions, the chances are you are shy. Shyness, again, takes different forms. There are those who hide behind the label of shy so that not too much will be expected of them. There are those who hate to be the centre of attention. Then there are those who love to be the centre of attention in a group, but are shy with one-to-one relationships. You only have to think of all

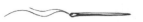

the famous actors and comedians who talk about being shy in their personal lives.

THE SHY SELF-PUBLICIST

One of my favourite American design heroes is a man credited with pioneering the field of industrial design in the United States: Raymond Loewy. He arrived in America from Europe without a penny to his name and knowing no-one, but went on to achieve enormous success. Loewy epitomizes the all-American dream. He became known for such American icons as The Greyhound bus, Air Force One, the Shell logos, the Nasa interiors for Skylab and the Space shuttle to name but a few. However, his success also lay in his genius for self-publicity. He did this by taking advantage of every possible opportunity to promote himself and his work.

Whenever he had his photograph taken, it was always posing in, on, or beside a Loewy designed product. Always impeccably dressed, he attended all the right social functions. He would throw lavish parties at his home for the most influential people. At dinner parties, he could always be relied on to entertain with charming and amusing anecdotes about his designs and the people he worked for. He was an excellent showman.

And yet, he was excruciatingly shy.

Loewy prepared ruthlessly for business meetings and presentations. Painstakingly, he would rehearse every word and joke to be used. He had a publicist who told him exactly what to say at interviews and he followed it to the letter. At social functions, Loewy's wife was not allowed to leave his side for fear he might be overcome with shyness and run out of things to say. He knew that in order to achieve the unusual, he had to do the unusual, and that is what he did. He loved the limelight, he wanted to be famous and successful, and he was prepared to work for it – overcoming his

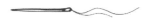

shyness was part of that. His shyness makes his achievements even more impressive.

Of course, it isn't necessary to go to such extremes but you do need to be prepared to make the effort, hard though it might be at first. You will know the form your shyness takes, think about it and know that you can help yourself. The Conroy Concept will help you.

Chapter Seven

You Deserve it and You can do it:
Using the Conroy Concept

You may have read something in the preceding chapter that resonates with how you think and feel. Hopefully, something that leads to your greater self-awareness. As a teenager researching self-esteem, I certainly recognized myself in some of what I read. Light bulbs flashed everywhere. I believe it was that new self-awareness that saved me from much unhappiness later on. Long before my self-awareness journey began (I know, journey is a much overused term but it is a word very much fit for purpose), a chance conversation with the headmistress at my school introduced me to alternative ways of thinking.

I was fifteen. My father had passed away but not before inflicting much suffering on his family during divorce proceedings. I was confused and angry. I loved school because I had fun there, too much fun. After an altercation with a teacher, I was sent to see the headmistress. Everyone feared Mrs Jackson (not her real name), even the other teachers. So, it was with some trepidation that I approached her office. I was about to knock on the door when it flew open and she growled, 'Inside and sit down!' With that she brushed past me out of the door. Tall, and dressed in full cap and gown she raced off down the corridor like Batman on a mission. Now, scared to death, I waited in her office for over an hour.

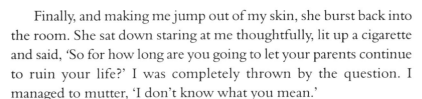

Finally, and making me jump out of my skin, she burst back into the room. She sat down staring at me thoughtfully, lit up a cigarette and said, 'So for how long are you going to let your parents continue to ruin your life?' I was completely thrown by the question. I managed to mutter, 'I don't know what you mean.'

We spent two hours together that day. She gave me tea, biscuits and tissues. I sobbed out everything that had been happening at home, some of which she already knew. Mrs Jackson explained to me that my parents had made bad choices in their lives and were now living with the consequences. The result of that was frustration, which led them to be impatient and quick to anger.

Despite my father's death, she felt he was still negatively affecting my behaviour. My mother, she said, was doing her best to bring up five children on her own but was frightened by that and bound to make mistakes. She told me none of that was my fault. However, in the next breath she told me what happened next in my life was entirely up to me. Explaining that, although I was very bright (I should have asked her to tell my Physics teacher), I was in danger of throwing it all away by allowing the situation at home to badly affect my schoolwork. If it continued, she said, I could kiss goodbye to a decent career. She also confided in me that she had been a 'latchkey kid' as a child. Often she and her sister would go for days without food and most evenings they could be found sitting on the steps of the local pub waiting for their parents to come out. She determined early on that her future would be better, and education was how she did it. If she could do it, so could I, is what she told me. I left her office thinking no-one would ever believe the conversation we had just had.

I wish I could tell you that I listened to Mrs Jackson and turned my life around. I didn't. At least, not then. I was too young and immature to fully understand. At that time, I saw my mother as totally dominant and couldn't imagine for a second that she was frightened by anything. I did listen when Mrs Jackson said that none

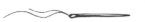

of what happened at home was my fault. My parent's behaviour towards me had more to do with them than it did with me. That part sunk in. Later, her words echoed down through my research and it was only then that I truly understood what she did for me that day.

I was in a home where, at times, the behaviour of the adults towards me was bewildering at best and cruel at worst. Children experiencing similar situations frequently think it must be their fault and blame themselves. This can lead to all kinds of issues later in life such as feelings of self-doubt and lack of worthiness, for example. Instead, for me, thanks to Mrs Jackson and my research into personal development, I found alternative understanding.

Everyone has a past. It's only when speaking openly and honestly to others about it that you begin to realize that most people have been through trials and tribulations of some sort. Whether it's because of negative experiences, parenting styles or even genetics, the causes may be argued elsewhere, you might find yourself at the mercy of SECS. It is what you are going to do about it next that counts.

You cannot continue all your life to blame your problems on your past or your parents. You need to look at the past but only in order to gain understanding. Question the past knowing what you know now. As an adult and a parent, I can look back at my father's behaviour, for example, and see his inadequacies. I wasn't equipped to do that as a child. Any beliefs formed about myself resulting from his behaviour then, were formed by the mind of a child and are false. Remember Mary? Different circumstances, same conversation. Identify any false beliefs and self-defeating patterns you may have and set about dismantling them. If you need professional help, get that too. For the moment, let's take another look at the Conroy Concept and see how it can be used to help solve your SECS problem.

Close relationships – Find a person whom you can trust and talk to them. Tell them how you feel. Confess to suffering from SECS. I know this isn't easy to do, especially if you have been successful at creating a false persona. Take a leap of faith. It will make your life a whole lot easier if you have a trusted ally on your side.

When I was a young woman and we were starting out in business, I met Alison, an older businesswoman whom I liked very much. We weren't in the same social circle but whenever we met, I enjoyed her company. She started inviting me to parties and various social gatherings but I always found a reason to decline. Every so often, I would receive an invitation and each time I made my excuses. The thought of having to socialize with her high-powered circle of older friends filled me with dread. I thought I would be out of my depth and would have nothing to say. I expected Alison would tire of me and stop sending invitations, but she didn't.

One afternoon I ran into her by accident, and we went for a coffee. As we stood to leave the coffee shop, she said, 'Oh, by the way, I'm having a dinner party at my home on Saturday, are you free to come?' In a split second I knew I couldn't make excuses. Responding with excuses on paper was one thing; lying to her face was quite another. Instead, I asked her to sit down again, took a deep breath and told her exactly how I felt. Apart from anything else, it was such a relief to be honest.

Alison was so generous with her words of encouragement and advice, telling me that she had been the same when she was younger. Social confidence, she assured me, would come with practice and maturity. I agreed to go to the dinner. For the rest of the week, the dinner hung over me like a dark cloud. I certainly wasn't looking forward to it.

On the night, Alison had arranged the seating so that I was right beside her. Although, I was uncomfortable at first, her support beside me was all I really needed. The other guests were delightful and I enjoyed the evening. The best part about this story is that Alison and I became much closer friends.

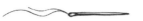

Demonstrating our own vulnerability allows others to do the same and that makes for a much more authentic friendship. After that, if I had to attend a function that might give me the jitters, as I call it, I would telephone Alison to talk it through.

EXERCISE 13:
TALK ABOUT IT

This week choose a close friend or family member whom you trust and schedule some time together for a chat. Maybe talk about a time where SECS caused you to act in a self-sabotaging way. Explain your thoughts and feelings to the person you have chosen. Open a discussion about it. You will feel so much better and it will also increase the other person's understanding of you. It might surprise you to hear that they too have examples of their own self-sabotaging behaviour. In this case, you can become each other's ally. Another baby step, but a step forward, nevertheless.

Outcome – Being outcome-focussed and goal-oriented. You already know that setting goals gives a strong sense of purpose. Reaching your goals gives you a strong sense of achievement. With each achievement, your confidence grows. As your confidence grows, you begin to like yourself more and yes, you've guessed it, that leads to an increase in self-esteem. There is no quicker way to increasing your self-esteem than seeing yourself succeed.

If you suffer from shyness, you could set yourself an overall goal to be more confident socially. What does that mean to you? Be specific.

The Vision – Imagine you are on this side of a river and across the other side there is a garden party happening. You can hear laughter and the clinking of glasses and children playing. You look across the river and all of a sudden you see yourself there at the party.

The person across the river is you having achieved your goal of being socially confident. How is that 'you' behaving? What are they doing differently to you as you are now? How are they standing? Are they noticeably relaxed? Perhaps they are chatting easily to someone. They might even be approaching a group and starting a conversation. Are they having fun? How does someone like you, who is shy, take such a huge leap to get from this side of the river to the other? You create stepping stones. The stepping stones are your goals. You have your overall vision; break it down now into easily manageable steps. Here are some examples:

Stepping stone 1. Learn to relax. There are many breathing techniques that will help you to relax. Practise these at length in the privacy of your own home. Soon you will be in a position where a few well timed deep breaths will quickly take you into a relaxed state. It will be easier for you to focus on your conversation if you are feeling calm. You will also appear to be more approachable to others than if you look tense and agitated.

Stepping stone 2. Practise your body language. When speaking to someone, do you stand up straight, with a relaxed, open stance and look them in the eye? Or, do you hold your head down with your body in a position set to run away? There are tons of books, videos and courses about how to use and understand body language. Sometimes altering your body language alone alters your state or the way you feel. Presenting confident, warm and friendly body language will draw people to you before you have even spoken.

Stepping stone 3. Learn communication skills. Yes, conversation is a skill. Some people are good at it, some people need more practice. That's all. Again, there is lots of information out there on this subject. You can even download conversation mind-maps that script conversations for various situations. You might think that sounds a

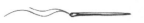

bit contrived but they are only a guide to get you started. Use them as a fall-back in a situation where you might run out of things to say. Scripting worked for Raymond Loewy, it might just work for you too.

The best advice I have ever been given in this regard is to remember that it's not all about you. Instead of worrying about how you are coming across or what you are going to say next, be interested in others. Be genuinely interested in others and what they have to say. Really listen. Listening is often more important than speaking. Why do you think you have two ears and only one mouth?

Stepping stone 4. Set tasks. Set yourself some small, safe and comfortable tasks to do to build your social confidence. For example, if eating alone in a restaurant bothers you, start by going for a coffee, stay for five minutes then leave. Next time stay for ten. Once that becomes easy, progress to another level.

Action Step – This is the most important step. Look at your stepping stones and choose one, two, or even three things you can do this week to get you closer to your vision.

1) Find a relaxation programme or technique that you think will work for you.
2) If you are feeling braver, begin a conversation with someone you haven't spoken to before, perhaps at work or some other safe environment. Think about what you might say beforehand and do it.
3) Set yourself a deadline by which you will have completed your action step.

Once you have completed your action steps, acknowledge and congratulate yourself. Finally, write your achievements down in your success journal (see below). Write about what happened and how you felt about it.

EXERCISE 14:
SUCCESS JOURNAL

Create a success journal. Everyone needs to do this. Write down everything you have ever achieved. Gather certificates and badges, pictures of your kids or your home. Include promotions or positive changes you've made. Write down everything you have ever done that you are proud of or that is important to you. Keep your journal close by where you can see it. Include a separate section for your goals. From now on, every time you achieve even the smallest thing, enter it in your journal. As you achieve each small goal, create another one a little more challenging than the last one and so on. Log them all down in your journal. You will soon begin to see that your achievements and your self-esteem grow mutually.

Now – Remember, this is about living in the now, being fully engaged in the present moment. It's about trying to stop thinking about the past or worrying about the future and, instead, focussing on the experience you are having right now. I talked about using a meditation practice to help you achieve this. I confess that I used to think of meditation as a way I could escape from the world for a while, hoping it would somehow help me to take a break from my current reality. I was mistaken. Meditation helps you to see reality differently or more clearly. When you begin to quieten the mind, of course, the mind wants to misbehave. It begins to wander. The secret is to be aware of the thoughts that appear, acknowledge them, and let them go. To watch your thoughts without becoming lost in them. Instead of being fully identified with them, you step out of your thoughts and learn to dissociate. If you remember, we talked about thoughts leading to feelings? If you can step back from negative thoughts and see them objectively as simply temporary events of the mind, you will have more control of your feelings. So

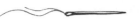

now a negative thought need not necessarily lead to a feeling of inadequacy, for example.

Recent studies in neurobiology have shown that this kind of mindful meditation can lead to permanent changes in the pre-frontal cortex area of the brain and the limbic systems, which are both involved in regulating the emotions.

I know there are some people who still think of meditation as some kind of 'flaky' activity that only religious or spiritual people do. If you are one of those, try instead to think of it as training of the mind. Training that helps you get closer to understanding the difference between the way things appear and the way they actually are. If you experience any level of SECS, meditation will help you to see your reality more clearly. It will allow you to change your relationship with your emotions, leading you to feel more comfortable with yourself. Once again, I would say that like any other kind of training, this takes time and effort. It is worth it.

Contribution – When you feel you are contributing to the greater good in whatever possible way, you feel better about yourself, of that there is no doubt. Volunteering your services free of charge to your community or to another person in any capacity has been shown time and again to help with SECS. In younger people, volunteering increases confidence. It instils a work ethic and a strong sense of accomplishment that leads them to understand their value to society. Older people who volunteer report significantly higher life satisfaction and fewer symptoms of depression and anxiety than those who don't volunteer. At any age, volunteering increases your social circle and improves social skills. Automatically, you have something in common with your fellow workers. Volunteering increases sense of purpose, achievement and self-worth.

Exercise – One summer during the school holidays, I finally took the children off to do something I had long been promising to do –

I took them rock climbing. My eldest son, Mitch, and I had climbed only once before when Josh and Charlotte were too young to join in. Since then Charlotte had her arm amputated. Now, all three children were asking to go climbing. It was a quandary. I didn't want the boys to miss out because their sister wouldn't be able to do it, and I didn't want to take the boys and leave Charlotte behind. We were acutely aware of the importance of building Charlotte's self-esteem at this time. Telling her there was something she couldn't do because of her arm went against everything we were trying to do for her. Eventually, I contacted the climbing guide and discussed it with him. He agreed that Charlotte should come too. I will leave you to imagine the practicalities of climbing with one hand only. Impossible? At this point, I must tell you that Robin does not like heights, and declined to join us for that reason. Charlotte had the choice to stay at home with Dad without feeling pressured to come along. She wouldn't hear of it.

So there we were. I was nervous for myself because I had struggled with climbing the first time, for Josh who was about eight years old, and for Charlotte with one arm. Mitch was the one about whom I was only marginally concerned. What a motley bunch. We had a distance to walk before we reached the climb site and all the way there Charlotte was encouraging me because she knew I was nervous.

We reached the rock and were kitted out and given instructions by the guide. The rock we were to climb was about forty feet high. Okay, I admit the height of this rock gets higher each time I tell the story, but it was much higher than our house, let's just say that.

Mitch went up first and was so graceful and strong, he made it look easy. I went next. I know it sounds a silly thing to say, but I was very quickly reminded of how 'rock hard' rock actually is. You know when you watch people climb on TV, you often see them gently swing into the rock and bounce back? Well, let me tell you, there is nothing gentle about it. That swinging into the rock hurts like the

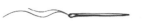

devil. So, my climb was complete with various grunting noises and yelps that had Charlotte and Josh rolling on the floor with laughter.

From below, I heard various directions shouted up by the guide about where to put my hands and feet next. In protest, I muttered various retorts such as, 'I can't reach that far.' And, 'I don't have that kind of strength.' With great effort, I finally reached the top and Mitch pulled me on to my stomach where I collapsed, exhausted but exhilarated.

Josh came up behind me in half the time, without the sound effects and with the joy of achievement shining in his eyes. Then it was Charlotte's turn.

The nature of this rock was such that it jutted out at the top in a way that meant you couldn't look over the edge and see down. The guide had told me that he was going to climb over Charlotte or around her like Spiderman. I was confident that she would be safe.

Now, the three of us waited for her at the top. We waited and waited. Occasionally, the guide shouted up, 'We're okay, she's doing fine.' We could hear him talking to Charlotte but we couldn't hear what they were saying.

Time went on and I became distraught. How could I put her through this? What was I trying to prove? That she was normal? Just like everybody else? All of these thoughts and more were going through my mind. Eventually, even the boys became concerned.

We heard them approaching the top and Charlotte's little face appeared over the edge of the rock. She was crying. Silent tears streaming down her face. Oh my goodness, what had I done? My heart lurched. I was about to burst into tears and shower her with apologies but the boys got to her first. They were jumping up and down with her shouting, 'You did it! You did it!' And Charlotte was laughing. She certainly went up in their estimation that day. You know, being a girl an' all. Being a girl with one hand and climbing up a forty foot rock took it to a whole different dimension. Quickly composed, instead of bursting into tears, I turned her around to look at the view from where we were standing and said, 'Just look at what you did. Look how high we are. Don't let anybody ever tell you there is something you cannot do because you have only one arm – *where there is a will, there is a way.*'

The guide was singing Charlotte's praises all the way back. When climbing with her, he assured her that any time she wanted to, they could easily abseil back down to the bottom and that would be fine. There was no way. It was grim determination that got her to the top. I didn't particularly like myself that day but I was so very proud of all three of my kids.

Looking back, I truly believe that experience helped to shape who Charlotte would become. That one achievement gave her the confidence to try. After that, we went gorge walking where she climbed up waterfalls. She went ice skating with her friends and took up horse riding again. One thing Charlotte declined to join in with was canoeing – she felt she would end up paddling round in circles… she had a sense of humour too.

The point of this story is to demonstrate that exercise or sport of any kind can be used as a tool to build confidence and self-esteem. The sense of achievement that climbing that rock gave to Charlotte made her feel so good about herself. It gave her confidence and self-esteem that transferred into other areas of her life.

CHOOSING THE BEST EXERCISE

As long ago as 1999 a study by the University of Bristol concluded that exercise is effective in reducing anxiety and improving self-esteem. Studies since corroborate their findings and offer further insights. The type of exercise or sport you take up is thought to be important if your goal is to improve self-esteem. For example, to begin with it might be a mistake to take up anything involving competition with others. The idea is to start with something where you can see yourself steadily improve. You need to be consistent, so choose something that you will enjoy as opposed to something you think you should do for quick results. Studies show, for example, that for older people Tai Chi is a good activity because it gently develops physical condition but also physical strength and body attractiveness, which leads to enhanced self-esteem. Younger people might enjoy the camaraderie of a team sport. Being part of a team means that winning and losing is shared.

One study demonstrated that self-esteem in overweight teenagers was enhanced through exercise even though they didn't actually lose weight. So it isn't only about exercising to lose weight or change body shape. It's about doing something good for yourself that you know is good for you in all kinds of ways. It is taking control and watching yourself get fitter.

In terms of the mood enhancing, feel good factor of exercising – weight training is good. Consistent, moderate aerobic intensity exercise is better than low intensity, e.g. walking, or higher intensity, e.g. hill running, which could increase anxiety.

Taking Charlotte climbing at such a sensitive time in her life was a very risky thing to do. What if she hadn't made it to the top and abseiled down instead? Would that have had an adverse effect on her feelings about herself? In the final analysis, I probably shouldn't have done it, but I will be forever thankful that I did.

Ironically, if you are depressed or suffer from SECS, the last thing you feel like doing is exercise. Motivate yourself by using pleasure (see below), choosing the right exercise for the right thing at the right time, and starting small. Remember:

'A journey of a thousand miles begins with one step.' (Lao Tzu)

Pleasure – Pleasure is not merely something nice to have now and then. It is something we all need. Suffering from SECS can be very stressful. Taking time to relax, have fun and be yourself is even more

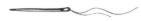

important for you. The exercise 'Digging for pleasure' in Chapter Four asks you to think of ten things that give you pleasure and to schedule them into your diary. I hope you did the exercise. Now I want you to dig even deeper and create a reward list.

Exercise 15:
REWARD LIST

This list, again, is of things that give you pleasure but this time, I want you to include some bigger and better things – luxury items, such as jewellery, handbags, a watch or new electronic gizmo. I love to stay in good hotels so my list here would include a night in a favourite hotel. You might enjoy massages or beauty treatments of some kind. Luxury items, but ones that you can afford or can easily save up for. You can have the items on your list but you must work for them. Each time you achieve something that takes you towards your goal of feeling better about yourself, for example, taking up some form of exercise, talking to that person, changing your way of thinking, or throwing that garden party – do something or buy yourself something from your reward list by way of congratulations. Use the items to motivate yourself to do something – 'I can have the handbag when I have… (you choose). When you finally get the handbag, the pleasure will be twofold. Once you have exhausted your reward list, and you will, make another one. How exciting is that?

Trying new things – Be open to trying something new. Specifically, learning something new. The research available demonstrating the positive effect that learning has on SECS is overwhelming. My favourite study is one carried out for The Centre for Research on the Wider Benefits of Learning in 2002. They surveyed 10,000 tutors. 92.5% of them agreed or strongly agreed that: 'Through their learning, my students on the whole experience improved self-

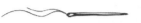
esteem.' Self-esteem and confidence are considered to be the most important benefits of further education, with developing a social network coming in closely behind. The suggested reasons given for this are course content, interaction between students, responsibility for own learning, and sense of purpose.

Learning is empowering. If you don't succeed at first, see that as research and learn from it, and experience your successes as confidence builders that will take you on to the next level.

Self-Awareness

My inclusion of chapters on the issue of SECS is not an attempt to address any deep emotional problems or to resolve deep issues with the past. It is an attempt to help you to use the Conroy Concept to create self-awareness, which I believe is the first step to creating your new understanding. Ultimately, I want that awareness to lead you to the new belief that, yes, you are worthy of happiness and, what's more, you deserve it. We all do.

Socrates said, 'Know thyself.' And, 'An unexamined life is not worth living.'

Benjamin Franklin said, 'There are three things extremely hard: steel, a diamond, and to know one's self.'

I agree with both men. Self-awareness isn't easy. It is an on-going process during which you will discover new things all the time. Each new thing you learn about yourself will give you the opportunity to change that thing if it doesn't serve you, and develop it if it does.

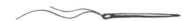

Chapter Eight

Uncover what Lies Beneath:
Discover your strengths and how to use them

N ow I want to talk about discovering and developing some new things about yourself that will serve you.

First, an exercise:

Exercise 16:
THINGS YOU DON'T AND THINGS YOU DO

Make sure you complete part a) before moving on to part b).

a)   Pick up your pen and quickly write down five things you do not like about yourself.
b)   Now write down five things you do like about yourself.

I would like to bet that it took you longer to write down the things you like about yourself than the ones you don't. Did you even get to five things you like? We are so quick to negatively judge ourselves and focus on what's wrong with us. It isn't only those with low self-esteem who are more willing to believe the failings in themselves; we all have a tendency to do it. Our brains are wired towards the negative. Even if we are told something good about ourselves, we often ignore it. Think of the last time you were paid a compliment. Did you respond by dismissing whatever it was, brushing it off as nothing? If I were to say five good things about you and one not so good, which one do you think you would focus on the most? When Socrates said 'know thyself', he wasn't just talking about your weaknesses. He was talking about the whole glorious you. Knowing thyself means being aware of your true self, your whole self, and that includes the good bits. It includes being aware of and acknowledging your strengths.

Before we talk about what I mean by strengths, let's take a quick look at why I include the subject in a book about helping yourself to happiness. Here are some of the ways you will benefit from becoming aware of your strengths and learning to play to them. You will:

- Be more confident
- Enhance your self-esteem
- Increase your levels of energy and vitality
- Decrease your stress levels
- Be more resilient
- Be more likely to achieve your goals
- Perform better at work
- Increase your happiness levels

There are a number of positive psychology studies to demonstrate the scientific underpinnings for each one of these statements. With such strong evidence showing such amazing benefits, I want you to add developing your strengths to your 'toolbox' for helping yourself to happiness.

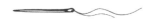

MANAGING WEAKNESSES

Most of us think that if we are to improve ourselves, we need to put all our attention on eradicating weaknesses. This is not surprising, as it's the way we have been brought up to think. All the way through our current education system, we are made aware of our weaknesses and encouraged to work on them. 'What's wrong with that?' you might ask.

Well, in education, for example, if you have a weakness in any area, it means you are less than 'average' at that particular subject. To use myself as an example, I was good at languages and, as you know, not so good at physics. Physics was a weakness I needed to address. This would have been difficult for me because I didn't enjoy the subject. I was never going to do very well at it. With effort, I could probably have pulled my test results around to average. This time and attention spent on physics would have been at the expense of spending time studying languages, thereby, decreasing my abilities in that subject. The end result would be that I was average at physics and average at languages.

That might be simplifying the case somewhat, but I think you understand my point. We end up with mediocrity in all areas instead of excellence in some.

I am not suggesting I should have ignored physics altogether. I am saying it would have been wrong to focus all of my attention on it, at the expense of other things. Transfer that story to personal development and what I am suggesting is that you manage your weaknesses, if you feel it necessary to do so. Some weaknesses don't even matter. Focus most of your attention on discovering and developing your strengths and create excellence in your life. I understand that this might be counter-intuitive to you, but I am not asking you take a leap of faith. As I said, the evidence speaks for itself.

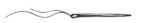

RECOGNIZING YOUR STRENGTHS

EXERCISE 17:
GIVE ME FIVE

A simple exercise. Write down your top five strengths.

Not so simple after all? It isn't simple because we are so unaccustomed to thinking about our strengths that we don't even have the language to do it. That is, not in any meaningful way. Your list might include things you are good at. Although you are most likely to be good at your strengths, your strengths do not include everything you are good at. For example, you might be brilliant at cleaning your house but hate doing it.

Your strengths are the natural positive traits you have that also make you feel good or strong when you engage in them. Your strengths strengthen you in every way. When you are using them you feel confident, uplifted and energised. Think about the last time you experienced the 'flow' situation we talked about in Chapter Four; a time when you were so absorbed in your activity you lost all track of time. The chances are you will have been engaging your strengths during that activity.

PATIENCE

Robin is a designer. As such, he often spends time with people helping them to make various design decisions. One day, a client arrived in the showroom to choose a door handle for his kitchen cabinets. An hour went by and the client made his choice, then changed his mind – three times. Finally, the choice was made and the client left. Robin was delighted with the choice. He felt it was

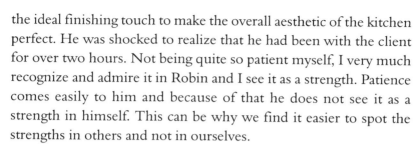

the ideal finishing touch to make the overall aesthetic of the kitchen perfect. He was shocked to realize that he had been with the client for over two hours. Not being quite so patient myself, I very much recognize and admire it in Robin and I see it as a strength. Patience comes easily to him and because of that he does not see it as a strength in himself. This can be why we find it easier to spot the strengths in others and not in ourselves.

You could try asking those around you what they see as your strengths and see if you agree with them. Or, you could take a more formal assessment. Over recent years there has been enormous interest and research into using a strengths approach in industry. Many organizations are coming to realize that their greatest potential is in the area of their greatest strengths. Organizations such as Aviva and Microsoft, to name but two, are seeing the benefits of becoming strength-based. There are now many strength assessment tools online. The one I prefer and suggest my students take is the scientifically validated VIA Inventory of Strengths (also known as the VIA Survey).

I prefer the VIA Survey because it sits very well alongside the Conroy Concept. It includes strengths that are valued across all cultures and religions and, whilst some assessments are designed to assess strengths pertinent to the workplace, the VIA Survey is one relevant to all areas of life, the professional, personal, and the spiritual.

The classification of strengths (VIA Classification) was developed by positive psychologists Christopher Peterson and Martin E. P. Seligman in 2004. This was completed after three years of research funded by the Mayerson Foundation, who offer the survey to be taken free of charge online. To date, over two million people from every country across the world have taken the test. The VIA Classification identifies six core virtues as headings that are then split into subheadings.

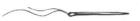

The result is twenty-four potential strengths:

1. **Wisdom and knowledge**. This refers to cognitive strengths involving learning and the use of knowledge.
    This category includes:
    a) Creativity: Thinking in original and productive ways.
    b) Curiosity: Being interested in experience for its own sake. Open to exploring and discovery.
    c) Judgement: Thinking things through, good critical thinking. Weighing evidence fairly.
    d) Love of Learning: Enjoying the mastery of new skills also related to the love of teaching others.
    e) Perspective: Having the ability to provide wisdom for others. Making sense of the world. Having wisdom.

2. **Courage.** Emotional strengths involving the use of will to achieve goals in the face of external or internal opposition.
    This category includes:
    a) Bravery: Standing up for your convictions. Facing up to threats, challenge, or difficulty. Not afraid to make unpopular decisions.
    b) Perseverance: Sticking with something. Finishing what you start. Not giving up in the face of obstacles.
    c) Honesty: Speaking the truth. Being genuine and authentic. Integrity.
    d) Zest: Feeling alive and filled with energy. Being activated and enthusiastic.

3. **Humanity.** Interpersonal strengths. Relationships with others.
    This category includes:
    a) Love: Valuing close relations with others.
    b) Kindness: Doing good deeds for others. Generosity and taking care of others.

    c)   Social Intelligence: Being aware of the feelings of others as well as your own. Knowing what makes others tick. Being able to fit into different social situations.

4. **Justice.** Strengths that help promote healthy community living. This category includes:
    a)   Teamwork: Social responsibility and loyalty. Working well as part of a team. Contributing to the group effort.
    b)   Fairness: Treating everyone the same. Not allowing personal feelings to bias decisions about others.
    c)   Leadership: Encouraging a group to produce the required result. Maintaining good relations with the group.

5. **Temperance**. Strengths that protect against excess. This category includes:
    a)   Forgiveness: Giving people a second chance. Not being vengeful.
    b)   Humility: Being humble in the face of your achievements. Modesty.
    c)   Prudence: Thinking carefully about your choices. Looking ahead. Being aware of consequences of actions.
    d)   Self-regulation: Being self-disciplined. Controlling your emotions and appetites.

6. **Transcendence**. Strengths that provide purpose and meaning. Connection with a larger universe. This category includes:
    a)   Appreciation of beauty and excellence: Experiencing awe and wonder. Noticing and appreciating beauty in different areas of life and the world.
    b)   Gratitude: Finding things to be thankful for.
    c)   Hope: Expecting the best from the future. Believing the future is good and working towards it.

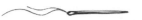

d) Humour: Seeing the light side of things. Laughter and playfulness.

e) Spirituality: Having faith and purpose. Belief about a higher purpose and the meaning of life. Connection to something larger than the self.

(This VIA Classification of six virtues and twenty-four character strengths was created by Peterson and Seligman (2004) and is copyright of the VIA Institute on Character (www.viacharacter.org). Used with permission. All rights reserved.)

Your top five strengths will be those you easily recognize in yourself, the ones that come most readily to you, and that make you feel the most energized when you use them. These are called your signature strengths.

EXERCISE 17:
GIVE ME FIVE – TAKE TWO

Now that you have read the VIA Classification of strengths, write down your top five strengths again.

An interesting addition to this exercise is to take the VIA Survey yourself, which you can do, as mentioned, free of charge at the VIA Institute online (www.viame.org/survey). Then compare the results with your own top five. The important thing to remember is that all twenty-four strengths are important and you will have them all in some measure.

The strengths that come at the bottom in your assessment are those that don't regularly occur as naturally for you. Strengths often overlap and support each other. You may also find that you use different strengths in different circumstances. The VIA Survey is an amazing descriptive tool that helps you to think about, consider and understand everything that is good about you as a human being. It gives you the language to be able to express what you learn about yourself, and it gives you something concrete to work with and build on.

Taking action with Strengths

The fun part now is learning how to use this new information to help yourself to more happiness. You could start by looking at your life on a daily basis to see how often you are using your top strengths.

Strengths at Work

My own top strength is love of learning. I spend much of my working day researching. It's why I love my job so much. Even in the car when traveling from A to B, I listen to personal development CDs. I am learning all the time. My second strength is curiosity and, here again, my work involves finding out about people and discovering different ways to help them. I find I perform at my best when I am able to use my top strengths, and you will too.

Balance is important. Sometimes, I can overdose on learning and so I am conscious of one of my other top strengths, which is appreciation of beauty and excellence. I am lucky enough to live in the countryside and I only have to walk outside to experience the most sensational view. My involvement with the art gallery also allows me to exercise this strength. If I haven't managed to visit a gallery for any length of time, I start to have withdrawal symptoms.

My other top strengths are perspective and honesty. Both are crucially important in my work. I am able to see the bigger picture and make practical sense of life. I am a good listener and know the right questions to ask to get results. Being honest is important for me professionally. However, this is a strength that can be a double-edged sword. Sometimes, I have to try to combine it with other strengths such as judgement and kindness. Being honest is also about being true to yourself. Being authentic. Have you ever said yes to someone, perhaps at work, when, in fact, you wanted to say no? Some people have a habit of doing that all the time. The consequence is that they never feel good about themselves.

Strengths at Play

Using your strengths will also help in your personal life. I mentioned that Robin and I have been married for over thirty years. I am often asked what I think is the secret to a happy marriage. Let me tell you a little story to demonstrate my answer. In our village, there is a little restaurant where Robin and I occasionally went for lunch. Even though we worked together, at that time, we often spent our days in different parts of the town visiting with clients. This meant we would each arrive at the restaurant separately. One day the owner of the restaurant, whom we had come to know quite well, told me, 'When you two first started to come in here we thought you must be having an affair.'

'Really?' I said. I couldn't imagine why.

'Yes,' she said, 'because you always arrive in separate cars and spend all lunchtime laughing and talking to each other.' A sad indictment on the institution of marriage.

So there are just two 'secrets' that I can tell you that help to keep my marriage happy. Using my strength of curiosity is the first. It helps me to stay interested and interesting, which I think is essential. Let's face it: boredom is the death knell to any relationship. The

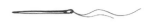

second secret is the use of humour, which features high on both of our strengths lists. You might now be thinking, 'Well, that's okay if curiosity is one of your strengths, but what if it isn't?' The beauty of working with character strengths is that you can find ways to foster them. So to develop your curiosity, for example, go back to the 'Try something new' section of the Concept for ideas. You could connect with a person from a different culture to your own and learn about that culture. I once went to a political meeting held by a Party I didn't vote for in an attempt to understand more. We talked about ways to foster humour in pleasure and fun (see page 56).

Spiritual Strengths

I went through a period where I knew I was neglecting the spiritual side of my life. I made the conscious decision to set time aside to devote to that. Reading a few lines of spiritual text every day brought me back to feeling centred. Whatever our particular term for it might be, regularly connecting to that which is larger than ourselves restores peaceful balance in our lives.

Strengths and Challenges

A good coach will work with you to help you utilize your core strengths in order to help you achieve your goals or solve any current problems. You might also feel you would like to develop some of your other strengths.

Using and developing your character strengths not only helps to increase your life satisfaction but it also helps you to blow away the black clouds, as I call them. Put another way, it helps you to overcome the obstacles and challenges in life.

Looking back at the experience of The Twilight zone with

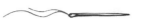

Charlotte and later with my sister Pat, I realize that, at some point or another, I harnessed every single one of the strengths listed in the VIA Survey.

Once Charlotte's arm had been amputated, she was monitored on a two-weekly basis to check whether or not the cancer had spread to her lungs. We later progressed to monthly and then three-monthly appointments. Given Charlotte's life expectancy of twelve months, you can imagine that the few days leading up to these appointments were filled with debilitating anxiety. It was faith, hope, love, bravery, kindness and honesty that we called upon. Later, when she needed to be fitted for a prosthetic arm, creativity, perseverance, perspective, humour and judgement were needed for sure. After much trial and error, Charlotte decided that a 'false' arm was not for her. Although, I disagreed with it, I had to exercise a certain amount of humility and put my own feelings aside and abide by her decision.

My sister further developed the strength of humility in me. Witnessing her astonishing bravery through every step of her devastating journey was incredibly humbling. She didn't take the VIA Survey but if I were to hazard a guess at her top strength, it would be bravery, followed closely by humour, perspective, social intelligence and perseverance. Being brave is not only about facing danger or extreme challenges; it is also about having the courage to stand up for yourself or to speak up when you think something is wrong.

STRENGTHS TO THE RESCUE

Dealing with health/medical services, for example (or any large organization), can be a daunting prospect. Most of the time, the people you deal with are lovely and are eager to help you. On the other hand, there are times when you feel that people and circumstances are purposefully collaborating to be objectionable.

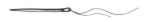

On these occasions, you may have to speak up to make yourself heard.

It doesn't always come easy. Remember, when you are ill, you are probably not operating at your best. If possible, it is always wise to have someone with you if you have to attend important hospital appointments. Whenever Pat and I were at an appointment, it was the consultant holding the meeting for whom I often felt sympathy. Having been through the system before, neither of us were afraid to ask for clarification if there was something we didn't understand. My 'curiosity' and Pat's 'persistence' sometimes meant the consultant was drilled, unmercifully, until Pat was satisfied that she had the knowledge she needed. In this particular instance, I wouldn't say that we enjoyed using our strengths but it was certainly empowering and it gave us the results we needed from that meeting.

Although my sister directed me to ask questions at meetings such as this (she believed that knowledge is power and it helped her to maintain some control over what was happening), I know there are others in the same circumstances who do not feel the same way. As I said before, always confirm that you have their permission before you ask questions on behalf of someone else.

Accessing your strengths to help you in times of adversity is much easier if you have already cultivated them beforehand. Knowing your own strengths and being able to draw on them will help you increase your happiness levels but will also allow you to operate at your best in any given circumstance.

Remember, 'know thyself' means know You – the whole you – the whole glorious you.

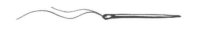

CHAPTER NINE

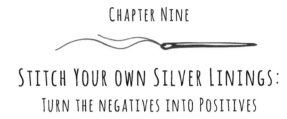

STITCH YOUR OWN SILVER LININGS:
TURN THE NEGATIVES INTO POSITIVES

THE CLOUDS

You now have the toolkit to put you in charge of your own happiness. Using just some of the ideas presented so far will increase the chances of success in your chosen career, your personal, financial, and your family life. Where I cannot guarantee blue skies and sunshine forever more in your life, I can guarantee you will be better equipped to deal with any cloud that threatens to rain on your parade.

Using the analogy of clouds, I often think of minor irritations as being the small white clouds that briefly block the sun, but soon pass by. Grey clouds are problems that need some attention, dark clouds are major challenges that take more effort to deal with, and black clouds are tragedies that, hopefully, don't come along too often.

THE NEEDLE

The Conroy Concept and its underpinnings, along with your strengths, combine to form the needle to help you stitch your own

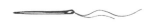

silver lining on any clouds that come your way. They give you the resilience you need to be more effective at dealing with even the blackest of clouds.

THE THREAD

Positivity is the thread to your needle. I am not talking here about forced positive thinking.

At an appointment with my sister one day, a nurse said to her, 'Now, remember, Pat, you have to stay positive.' Pat replied, with tongue firmly in cheek, 'Oh yes, I am very positive,' and whispered to me, 'Very positively dying.' She was terminally ill – telling her to 'stay positive' was almost insulting. We heard it so many times and mostly Pat would roll her eyes at me and smile. Some people mean well by it but, all too often, it's a platitude thrown out when they can't think of anything else to say. Thinking positively has its place, but not here. Here, I am talking about genuinely feeling and acting positive. As it happens, my sister was the most genuinely positive, terminally ill person you could ever meet. Of course, she had the benefit of the Conroy Concept – much of which she helped to develop.

So how do you make the transition from forced or fake 'positive thinking' to genuinely feeling positive? Allow me to remind you of our definition of happiness.

'Living a flourishing and fulfilling life, experiencing positive emotions most of the time.'

Let's investigate these positive emotions. According to leading, positive psychologist Barbara Fredrickson in her ground-breaking book, *Positivity* (2010), the following are the top ten positive emotions accompanied by my own interpretations:

Joy – Thrilling moments.
It isn't a word in common use any more, is it? Yet, everybody

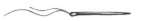

knows how it feels. It's when you have a thrilling moment that completely lifts your soul. What brings you joy?

Momentous occasions in my life such as giving birth and getting married brought joy to me. Another of my most thrilling and joyous moments was opening the letter that told me I had graduated from my Art and Design History degree with First class honours. Actually, I was overjoyed. There were butterflies fluttering around my whole body on that day. Before Mum passed away, I promised her that I would graduate and I would do so with First class honours. I worked conscientiously to make sure it happened.

Gratitude – Appreciation, whichever you prefer. We talked about this in Chapter Five.

Serenity – A sense of quiet peacefulness.

In the early evening, after a successful day and half an hour of meditation, I often sit outside in my back garden (admiring my stone walls) feeling a sense of quiet serenity. Do you ever have the feeling that right now, in this present moment, all is well with your world? It might be fleeting but if you recognize the feeling and nurture it, you can prolong it.

Interest – Doing something that captures your attention and eager engagement.

As described in 'Trying something new' (the 'T' in the Concept, see page 63), interest gives you purpose and intention.

Hope – A belief that things can be better.

Hope comes about when there is something you want or need to happen that isn't happening already. It happens when you are uncertain about an outcome. Hope gave me strength through all of the Conroy women's illnesses. It is a belief that things can change for the better, that there is light at the end of the tunnel.

Pride – Satisfaction brought about by achievement.

Not pride of the seven deadly sin variety, meaning someone who has an excessively high opinion of themselves. This pride is referring to that lovely feeling of satisfaction felt after an achievement of some kind. It can be an achievement by your country, your friends and family, or your own. Putting effort into something that brings about a successful result is a wonderful feeling. If the achievement is witnessed and acknowledged by others, it can be even better. That's why we often want to say, 'Look at what I did.'

The achievement doesn't have to be big. A simple example: I feel a sense of pride every time I water my houseplants. I have never been that successful with houseplants. However, for my birthday five years ago, a friend gave me a beautiful plant that still thrives today. I am so proud of it. I feel much more satisfaction when someone comments on that one than on any other. To feel this sense of pride regularly, you need to become practised at recognizing and giving yourself credit for your achievements, however small they might be. Your success journal will help with this.

Yes, pride running unchecked can result in the 'seventh deadly sin' meaning, but for most of us taking pride in our achievements is a positive emotion.

Amusement – Big enjoyable belly laughs.

It's also about the little things that happen, hopefully, many times over the course of the day. A wry comment somebody makes that brings out a smile, something silly your children do, sharing a joke with the ones you love. A light moment that lifts your mood.

Inspiration – Someone or something that gives you an irresistibly strong urge to do something creative, different or new.

The women in my life inspired me to put the Conroy Concept down on paper. They inspired me to want to help as many people as possible to increase the enjoyment in their lives.

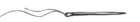

If ever I feel in need of some quick inspiration, I read Nelson Mandela's inaugural speech from 1994, written by Marianne Williamson. I suggest you do the same. On a more practical level, I love fashion and interior design magazines. They inspire me to try a new style of dress or be bolder with colour when redecorating my home.

Awe – Becoming overwhelmed by a sense of wonder.

Nature often does this for me. I can recall many times when I have been caught 'having a moment', as my kids call it.

We live in the countryside in the North of England and the sky is big but often too cloudy to see many stars. One year, we were on holiday in Yosemite National Park in the United States. We were outside on the balcony of our chalet as night fell. There were so many stars crammed into the sky and so close that it felt like we could reach out and touch them. Never having seen anything like it before, we lay on our backs stargazing for hours. I was so awestruck it brought me to tears.

Awe is that awareness of something larger that makes you feel small and humble on the one hand, yet very much a part of something extraordinary on the other. I am always on the look-out for this experience and can find it even in a single flower. To feel a sense of wonder like this in even the smallest of things you must slow down and practise the 'N' of the Concept, living in the 'Now', otherwise you miss what's right in front of you.

Love – The strongest, the king or queen of emotions.

This is an emotion that we would even die for. It nourishes the soul and gives reason to live. It can include all of the other emotions. Indeed, when we are 'in love' our capacity to experience all the other emotions increases. What is love? Well there have been numerous poets throughout time who have written about it and with whom I wouldn't dream of trying to compete. I do like this simple definition by the American author Oliver Wendell Holmes: 'Love is the master

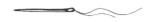

key that opens the gates of happiness.'

If you feel any of these emotions are in short supply for you right now, or if only to be certain that you are regularly experiencing them all, try the following exercise:

EXERCISE 18:
DEVELOPING YOUR POSITIVE EMOTIONS (PEMS)

Each week choose one of the following:

- joy
- gratitude
- serenity
- interest
- hope
- pride
- amusement
- inspiration
- awe
- love

Let's say you choose serenity. Write the word in big letters on a coloured 'sticky' note and stick it on your bathroom mirror, on your computer, or somewhere you will see it as a reminder every day. Think of different ways you can deliberately foster serenity. For example, schedule ten minutes at lunchtime to take a break from work and walk through a park. Sit alone somewhere and enjoy nature. Or, sit in meditation for a while. Go to an art gallery; they can be incredibly peaceful places to be. Do something each day of the week to give you that sense of calm and peace.

Some emotions are more difficult to cultivate than others. Use your imagination. You can see it as a challenge which will, in itself, pique your interest. Make it your business to practise these positive emotions most of the time until experiencing them begins to happen naturally.

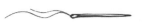

Broaden and Build Theory

It feels good to feel good, but positivity is about much more than that. I have said that negative emotions have their place by, for example, alerting danger. When faced with danger, negativity such as fear narrows your thinking and actions to allow you to focus on eliminating the threat. It's a much needed survival instinct. Positive emotions, on the other hand, according to Barbara Fredrickson, broaden your thinking and actions by making you more open and creative. They help to build knowledge and understanding that can help in future situations.

Experiencing positive emotions indirectly prepares you for dealing with trying times in the future. Research tests this by exploring how experiencing positive emotions changes the way people think and behave.

The better it gets, the better it gets. Positivity begets positivity. If you are interested, you are more likely to feel a sense of awe followed by serenity. If you feel love, you are more likely to feel gratitude. You become open to feeling good, which increases your positivity ratio and leads to an upward spiral of thriving.

Tipping point

How much positivity does one person need? In collaboration with social and organizational psychologist Marcial Losada, Fredrickson's research on positive emotions was translated into a mathematical equation. Accordingly, there is a 3:1 tipping point. Anything below that ratio of feeling three positive emotions for every one negative emotion creates a state of languish, where you are lacking vitality and enthusiasm for life. Anything above that ratio propels you into flourishing or thriving, which is what we are aiming for. Since the Losada/Fredrickson collaboration,

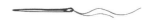

research carried out by scientists all over the world supports these findings.

When you think about it, bad feelings are stronger than good feelings. The idea that you need three positive emotions to balance one negative makes sense. Again, concrete findings that give us more to work with. If you want to thrive, you need to be feeling a ratio of at least four positive emotions for every negative. This is over time and in general, not necessarily on any given day.

EMBRACE EVERYDAY PROBLEMS AND CONCERNS

Some days, those I call blanket grey cloud days, are filled with one problem after another and positive emotions are few and far between. Occasionally, you might have dark cloud days – those with bigger issues and concerns. Try to reframe your thinking about them. Welcome problems as positive opportunities for development. Thread some humour into the situation. Be interested in how to resolve the problem. Maybe be inspired by how someone else has approached a similar situation. You will be amazed at the difference having this approach makes to your success at solving issues. Whether or not you are aware of it, you will become a better person as a result of successfully dealing with difficulties. Purposefully recognizing the fact softens the blow of a hard day. Problems can sometimes be positive.

When I was about fifteen, I remember Mum quizzing me about a falling out I had with one of my friends. I described my friend to Mum as being 'empty' and said I didn't want to be friends with her anymore. I wasn't even sure what I meant by that. My friend, Elizabeth (not her real name), came from a comparatively happy and comfortable home. She was a pleasant girl but had little to say and never seemed to want to do anything except tag along. She came from a loving home and, as the youngest of four children, was given pretty much whatever she wanted. She always wore fashionable clothes, had extra money to spend and never did anything to get into trouble. Nothing went wrong in Elizabeth's life.

Remember, I was a rebel. My father had died, but not before he had caused us untold misery. At that time, my mother was hard and controlling. We never had any money and I was always in trouble. I was Elizabeth's friend because I felt sorry for her. I felt sorry for her. I know now that when I described Elizabeth as *'empty'*, I meant shallow. In those days, she was shallow, but it wasn't her fault.

The problem with Elizabeth was she never had any. There were no ups and downs in her world. She lived life on an even keel. Although I couldn't articulate it properly, I did have some understanding of what was wrong. I expressed it at that time by saying she was boring. I was very young.

Elizabeth will, no doubt, have gone on to face problems in her life. I hope not too many and I hope she was equipped to deal with them. I believe it was dealing with adversity in my own childhood that helped me to develop qualities that, later, marched up alongside me just when they were needed: qualities such as stubbornness and defiance, yes, but willpower too, along with understanding and, of course, character strengths.

It could be argued that, at fourteen, life should be plain sailing, that depth and strength of character can wait until later to be built. I agree. There has to be better ways to build those qualities without having to suffer through a childhood like mine. Yet, I know that if you want to become a better person and gain more enjoyment from your life, you need to encounter a certain amount of hardship in your life. Welcome it when it comes. You will appreciate the sun much more after the occasional rain shower and, remember, a flower needs both to come into full bloom.

Whether you are facing grey cloud problems, dark or even black clouds, there is one final thing to help you break through them faster. Find the positive in the negative. Find something good from the bad things that happen to you.

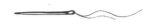

THE LESSON

When Robin and I lost the family business, we were devastated. Still, it taught us valuable lessons that we were able to draw on when we went on to start a new business. For example, Robin learned that he didn't have to shoulder all his business concerns by himself, which is what he had tried to do. He learned that by finding the right people to talk to he could find the right solutions. We chose to learn from a bad experience and so found a positive purpose for its happening.

Sometimes an experience is so bad there is nothing good to come out of it, except a lesson learned. Ask yourself right there and then as things are going wrong, 'What is the lesson here?' The lesson itself can often give you the answer to help you move forward. Learning it stops you from making the same mistake again.

THE GIFT

So many times in my spiritual and personal development studies, I heard it said, 'Look for the gift.' Look for the gift in any difficult or tragic experience. I confess to finding it a difficult thing to say to others I meet who are experiencing challenging times. I never say it lightly, and timing is important but I do, gently, persist. I know there is always a gift.

Without doubt my experiences with Charlotte made me a better person. I became much more aware of the suffering of others. Compassion became a strength. I developed empathy and understanding. Actually, if I'm honest, it also fostered a lack of patience in me. I am now impatient with small mindedness and insincerity. My strength of honesty includes a need for authenticity both in myself and those I deal with. I am less inclined to accept injustice and more inclined to be assertive than before. These were

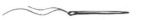

important, positive behaviour changes for me. I developed a strong spiritual practice and am much more appreciative of everything and everybody in my life.

The gift of my sister Pat's cancer, as with my mum's, was time. Time to say all the things we wanted and needed to say to each other. Pat's illness opened up conversations between us that were about much more than saying 'I love you'. They were deep and soulful conversations. Unspeakable conversations where we struggled to express thoughts and emotions. They were emotions we had never felt before or even understood. We were often forced to think very carefully, to dig deep and speak from the heart. These conversations were a gift for me because they took our relationship to a much greater closeness and depth of understanding. Such raw honesty and openness would not have taken place under any other circumstances; there would be no need. I cherish those times.

After surviving the first attack of lymphoma, Pat searched for purpose and meaning in her experience. What was her gift from it? She couldn't immediately see a purpose to it so she made one. Something her consultant oncologist lamented about his job was that, because of time constraints, he often found himself delivering the 'Sorry, it's cancer' news to someone and having to leave them to deal with it alone. Ideally, he wished for a qualified counsellor or trained member of staff to follow behind him and spend time with his patient. If the money could be raised to fund a twelve month salary for someone, there was a possibility that the position would become permanent.

Pat made this her purpose. She went on to raise £35,000, which at the time was more than enough to pay a salary. Now that's what I call making a positive from a negative.

The lessons and the gifts are the silver linings for your clouds.

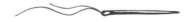

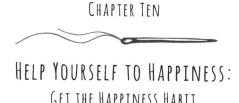

CHAPTER TEN

HELP YOURSELF TO HAPPINESS:
GET THE HAPPINESS HABIT

Now you know what makes you happy, how to be happy, and how to stay that way, most of the time. Your circumstances may change but you will have a foundation in place that will remain unshaken. From this foundation you can go on to build your own version of success. As I told my son who started to live his life the Conroy Concept way:

'Now, you can have your red Ferrari in the drive. Now, you can have a large house and expensive things; if that's what you want. You can enjoy your possessions but you won't rely on them to make you happy. If you achieve material wealth and, as happened to us, lose it all – your happiness and well-being will not be affected.'

You can be confident now that you have the strength and resilience to start again, in whatever way you choose.

Remember the important things you need to accept:

YOU NEED OTHER PEOPLE

We all do. Take time to nurture your existing relationships and make new ones. If you have some relationships that are, what I call, 'toxic', where time spent with the person leaves you feeling drained or upset, try talking to them about it. Explain how you feel. Find out if there is something good between you worth salvaging. If you have tried everything you can and it makes little difference, it might be better for both of you if you gently release your relationship. Wish them well and move on.

Open up your heart to those around you, be honest and sometimes vulnerable. Ask for help when you need it. There are no problems you are facing that someone hasn't faced before you. Therefore, there must be someone who can help you. Equally, you will have the experience to help others in the same way. Don't allow a few minutes of possible discomfort to stop you being there for a friend in need.

YOU NEED A VISION

You need a vision for your own life. Not a vision you feel you should have or a vision that someone else has for you. You must decide what you want, understand what needs to be done to get it and take action. Have a plan. Be outcome-oriented and set goals. You don't even need to know all the steps you need to take. Often its only when you take the first step that your second step becomes obvious.

I love the analogy of driving your car in thick fog. You may only be able to see a hundred yards in front of you, but by driving slowly and thoughtfully, you move forward until you can see the next hundred yards, and then the next. You just keep going until you reach your destination.

Apply this way of thinking to all areas of your life. There will be obstacles along the way. There is no such thing as a problem-free life, but when problems do come along, you can control how to deal with them. Change the way you think about your problems. They are essential to help us learn and grow. When we stop growing, we 'rot'. Just because it's a cliché to say 'think of problems as obstacles' doesn't make doing so any less effective. Make your thinking work for you. Find the learning and the gifts and turn negatives into positives.

STILLNESS AND SILENCE

Stop running around busying yourself so much. Take a breath. Ask yourself why you feel the need to be busy all the time. Is it because you are avoiding something? Your feelings, for example? Spend some quiet time becoming aware of yourself. Take a moment to check in with how you are feeling. Notice your 'negative self-talk' thoughts and question them. Run them through the 'thinging' test and remember, simply because you are thinking something doesn't make it true.

A meditation practice will help you learn to engage with and enjoy what's happening to you right at this moment. The present moment. Meditation will help you to tune in to your own needs. Listen to your intuition and take your own counsel. You have all the answers, but you must be still and silent long enough to hear them.

YOU CAN MAKE A DIFFERENCE

Watching the nightly news on TV can often make one feel helpless and overwhelmed by the world and its problems. You cannot solve all of the world's problems but then, you don't have to. You only have to help one person right now and cause the ripple effect.

Think about your strengths and the things you enjoy doing and find a way to harness them to help a deserving organization or society. If you can't spare the time but can afford to tithe money, choose a group whom you feel do good work and help them financially. If you don't have the time or the money, just smile at people, open doors for them, say thank you. Cheer up somebody's day – it will make all the difference.

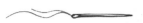

YOUR BODY NEEDS YOU

Look after that body that serves you relentlessly every single day. Nourish it with good food. Drink plenty of water (I am getting better), and take plenty of rest and exercise. You could live to be a hundred years or more. You need your body to be in good working order to help you make the most of all that glorious time on earth.

THE GOOD THINGS IN LIFE

That is pleasure and fun. Deliberately take time to create them in your life. If, like most people in the Western world, you work too hard for too long, you will become jaded. If you become jaded, you cannot perform at your best. That applies whether you are a chief executive or a stay-at-home mum. Especially if you are caring for someone who is sick, indulging in pleasure and fun little and often will keep you refreshed, vital, and on purpose. Never feel guilty for taking time out for yourself. You need it if you are to be of any help to those around you.

IF YOU DON'T USE IT, YOU LOSE IT

Continue to find different ways to use your brain. Challenge yourself at every opportunity. To make the most of learning you need to actively engage with whatever you are doing. That means more than passively listening to a lecture, or watching a TV documentary, for example, but questioning and deepening your understanding of the material. The sad fact is that ten minutes after listening to a talk, for example, you will probably remember only about thirty percent of its content. So, take notes, ask questions, and talk about what you have learned. If you get the opportunity to put into practice what you have learned, that's even better. Using this two-pronged attack, learning followed by putting it into practice gives your brain the best opportunity to create new neural pathways to allow it to grow.

ENJOY YOUR LIFE

I believe we are put on this earth to enjoy it. All of us. Jesus said:
'I came that you may have and enjoy life and have it in abundance, until it overflows.'
By 'you' he means everyone. Everyone deserves to be happy.
In the wider sense, I know the challenges are eradicating poverty and finding ways to live together harmoniously. I see evidence every day of people helping others to do just that, despite what the evening news tells us. We may have some way to go, but if all of us 'be the change we want to see', it will happen.
Start by increasing your own happiness and well-being. You are a work in progress. Seek out new information and ask, 'How can I use that in my life?' Explore spiritual teachings. Take full advantage of all the new scientific discoveries. Read books, take classes.
Be patient with yourself. Forming new habits is about repetition. When you start anything new, it feels strange, even difficult. With repetition it becomes easier. Once you find something is easy, you start to enjoy it, which leads to your wanting to do more. Before you know it, you will have formed a new habit. The Happiness Habit. Always keep in mind that you are in control of your own life.
You can stitch your own silver linings on every cloud and you can help yourself to happiness.

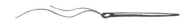

...AND FINALLY

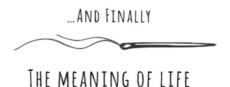

THE MEANING OF LIFE

C ancer has featured heavily in my life and those around me. Before long it is going to feature somewhat in the lives of everyone. In April 2011 Cancer Research UK reported that one in three people will develop some form of cancer at some time in their lives. A grim statistic indeed. A cancer diagnosis not only affects the patient, it affects everyone around them. It will touch us all.

However, predictions are already being made that twenty years down the line, cancer will be seen as a chronic illness that can be prevented or controlled. Eventually, according to Professor Sikora, leading cancer specialist at the University of Buckingham, a diagnosis of cancer will not be something to fear. This is absolutely fantastic news.

Even today many of the cancers that were once killers are treatable.

For my mother, sister and daughter the diagnosis of cancer was earth-shattering. With every fibre of my being I wish I could have changed that. I couldn't. What I could do was everything in my power to help them navigate their way through their situations as lightly and with as much grace as possible.

If you have lost someone you love, I am so very deeply sorry. I understand how totally debilitating it is. You must give yourself time to go through the natural process of grieving. By that, I mean your

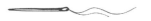

own natural process of grieving. We are all different. Go through the process in your own good time and be gentle with yourself.

After that you have a choice. You can allow the passing of your loved one to negatively affect your life by becoming bitter, self-pitying and lacking in purpose. Or, you can find a way to honour them. You can use the depth of your feelings to strengthen your resolve to live the rest of your life in a richer, more rewarding and fulfilling way. Which do you think your loved one would want for you?

For me, it is important not to allow the suffering of my Conroy Women to be in vain. I feel I owe it to them to enjoy and savour every minute of the time I have left. I decided to use what happened to them to help ease the path for others suffering in similar ways. I can learn from their experiences and make them mean something.

What is the meaning of life? Whatever meaning you choose to give it.

MY HEROES

Mum passed away just before the dawn of the new millennium. She was ready. She had brought up five children almost singlehandedly and sometimes under extreme and difficult financial conditions. Someone who didn't know better might think that, because of her struggles, she must have had an unhappy life. They would be wrong. Mum loved her children and her fourteen grandchildren and took great interest and joy in everything we did. We loved her dearly. She was happy.

Once, prompted by a drama on TV where there was fighting amongst a family about their father's will, she said to me, 'Well, at least, I know there will be no fighting over my will. I have nothing to leave you.' That's where she was wrong. What she left me is worth far more than anything she could have left me from 'her

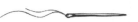

estate'. She left me her strength, her schoolgirl sense of humour, and a practical wisdom I draw upon every day. She is my inspiration.

When writing about Pat towards the end of the book, you may have noticed I began to use the past tense. At forty-six years old, after enduring cancer on and off for over twenty-five years, my beautiful, beautiful sister was finally released from suffering. She passed away, leaving those of us behind bereft without her. She contributed to the Conroy Concept of Happiness and encouraged me from the beginning. I promised her I would not allow grief to stop me from writing. She wanted me to tell those of you who may have been diagnosed with cancer not to allow it to make you a victim. Instead, use it as a wake-up call to change anything about your life you don't like. Live each day in the moment and learn to appreciate everything.

Something she did was to set about contacting the people from her past to say things she felt had been left unsaid. It was a brave and inspiring thing to see. When her time to leave us came, her family was around her bed. We sat through the night with her, holding her in turn – listening to her favourite music, laughing and talking together.

With all of my experience, my education, and research into the human condition; with all of my spiritual endeavours; I still cannot fathom my sister's absence. She was alive and vital and now she is nowhere to be seen.

I am working back through some of the Conroy Concept myself right now, and I confess to finding it a daily struggle. At times, I miss my baby sister, who became my best friend, with such ferocity it renders me too weak to walk. Pat was the bravest, funniest and most positive person I have ever known. I am honoured to be her sister. I know there will come a time when I am able to remember her, not with tears but with joy in my heart and a smile on my face.

In the meantime, it helps me to remember those words of wisdom spoken years ago by my seven year old daughter:

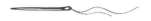

'Never mind, I will probably get used to it tomorrow.'

Speaking of my daughter. The one who, all those years ago, was herself given only twelve months to live? We got to celebrate her twenty-first birthday after all. Charlotte is now a gorgeous young woman and full of life. She works helping young people who are challenged in some way, either physically, mentally or socially. She is strong and brave, practical and positive, funny and inspirational.

I think she gets it from her mum's side.

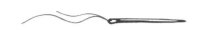

BIBLIOGRAPHY

Berne, E. (1966) *Games People Play: The Psychology of Human Relationships.* London: Penguin

Biswas-Diener, R. & Dean, B. (2007) *Positive Psychology Coaching: Putting the Science of Happiness to Work for Your Clients.* New Jersey: John Wiley and Sons

Biswas-Diener, R. (2013) *Invitation to Positive Psychology: Research and Tools for the Professional.* CAPP Press

Boniwell, I. (2006) *Positive Psychology in a Nutshell.* London: PWBC

Craig, C. (2006) *Positive Psychology Resources: Confidence.* Available at: www.centreforconfidence.co.uk

Branden, Nathaniel (2001) *The Psychology of Self-Esteem.* San Francisco: Jossey Bass

Dispenza, Joe D.C. (2007) *Evolve Your Brain: The Science of Changing Your Mind.* Florida: Health Communications, Inc.

Emler, N. (2001) *The Costs and Causes of Low Self-Esteem.* UK: Joseph Rowntree Foundation.

Emmons, A. Robert, Ph.D. (2008) *Thanks! How Practicing Gratitude Can Make You Happier.* New York: Houghton Mifflin

Frankl, Viktor E. (2004) *Man's Search For Meaning: The classic tribute to hope from the Holocaust.* London: Rider

Fredrickson, B. (2009) *Positivity Portfolio.* PowerPoint presentation for IPPA First World Congress of Positive Psychology. Philadelphia

Fredrickson, B. (2010) *Positivity: Groundbreaking Research to Release your Inner Optimist and Thrive.* Oxford: One World Publications

Friedman, M. (2012) *Art Can Be Good for Mental Health.* Available at: www.huffingtonpostcom/michael-friedman-lmsw

Gilhooly, M. Prof. (2007) *Flourishing in Older Age: Scottish and other realities (positive ageing).* PowerPoint presentation for Centre for Confidence and Well-Being.

Harris, T. A. (2012) *I'm OK, You're OK.* London: Arrow

Holmes, A. (2013) *Oldest People from Britain. Oldest Person in the UK: Grace Jones.* Available at: http://oldestinbritain.nfshost.com

Ivtzan, I., Gardner, H. E., & Smailova, Z., (2011) *Mindfulness meditation and curiosity: The contributing factors to wellbeing and the process of closing the self-discrepancy gap.* International Journal of Wellbeing, 1(3), 316-326. doi:10.5502/ijw.v1i22

Kristof, K.M. (2005) *Money Can't Buy Happiness, Security Either.* Available at: http://articles.latimes.com/2005/jan/14/business/fi-richpoll14

Kelly, R. (2010) *Changing Limiting Beliefs: Create all the health, happiness and success that you really want.* England: Rob Kelly Publishing

Lyubomirsky, S., King, L., Diener, E. (2005) *The Benefits of Frequent Positive Affect: Does Happiness Lead to Success?* Psychological Bulletin vol. 131, No. 6, pp. 803-855

Lyubomirsky, S. (2007) *The How of Happiness. A Practical Guide to Getting the Life You Want.* Great Britain: Sphere

Lyubomirsky, S. (2009) *The How, What, When, and Why of Happiness: Mechanisms Underlying the Success of Positive Interventions.* PowerPoint presentation for IPPA First world Congress of Positive Psychology. Philadelphia

Linley, A. (2008) *Average to A+ Realising Strengths in Yourself and Others.* United Kingdom: CAPP Press

Mountain Dreamer, Oriah. (1999) *The Invitation.* London: Harper Collins

Niemiec, R. (2012) *Mindful living: Character strengths interventions as pathways for the five mindfulness trainings.* International Journal of Wellbeing, 2(1), 22–33. doi:10.5502/ijw.v2i1.2

Peale, N. V. (1953) *The Power of Positive Thinking.* Great Britain: Vermillion

Peterson, C (2006) *A Primer in Positive Psychology.* New York: Oxford University Press

Peterson, C., & Park, N. (2009) *Classifying and Measuring Strengths of Character.* In *Oxford Handbook of Positive Psychology*, 2nd edition (pp. 25-33). New York: Oxford University Press

Peterson, C., & Seligman, M.E.P. (2004) *Character Strengths and Virtues: A handbook and classification.* New York: Oxford University Press and Washington, DC: American Psychological Association

Pink, Daniel H. (2008) *A Whole New Mind: Why Right-Brainers Will Rule the Future.* Great Britain: Marshall Cavendish Limited

Preston, J. and Hammond, C. (2002) *The Wider Benefits of Further Education: Practitioner Views.* London: The Centre for Research on the Wider Benefits of Learning Institute of Education

Ricard, Matthieu (2008) *Why Meditate: Working with Thoughts and Emotions.* Paris: Nil Editions

Ricard, M. (2011) The Dalai Lama: Happiness From Within. *International Journal of Wellbeing,* 1 (2), 274-290. doi:10.5502/ijw.v1i2.9

Seligman, Martin E.P. Ph.D. (2006) *Learned Optimism: How to Change Your Mind and Your Life.* New York: Vintage Books

Seligman, Martin E.P. Ph.D. (2007) *What You Can Change... And What You Can't: The Complete Guide to Successful Self-Improvement.* London: Nicholas Brealey

Schonberger, A. (ed.) (1995) *Raymond Loewy: Pioneer of American Industrial Design.* New York: Prestel

Shwader, Marilyn (ed.) (2002) *A Guide to Getting It: Self Esteem.* Portland, Oregon: Clarity of Vision Publishing

Sorensen, Marilyn J. Ph.D (2006) *Breaking the Chain of Low Self-Esteem.* Tigard, Or: Wolf Publishing Co.

Sikora, K. (2009) *Soon We Won't Have to Fear Cancer.* Available at The Telegraph: www.telegraph.co.uk/health/5045618/Soon-we-wont-have-to-fear-cancer.html

Dianne, R.& Grant Anthony, M. (ed.) (2006) *Evidence Based Coaching Handbook.* New Jersey: John Wiley and Sons

Tayyab, R. (n.d.) *340 Ways.* Available at: http://tayyabrashid.com/pdf/via_strengths.pdf

Peggy, A., Hewitt Lyndi N. (2001) *Volunteer Work and Wellbeing.* Journal of Health and Social Behavior, 2001, Vol 42, (June): 115–31

Tracy, Brian. (n.d.) *Twelve Step Goal Setting Process.* Available at: http://media.briantracy.com/downloads/pdf/12stepgoalsettingpr ocess.pdf

Tugade, M. M., Fredrickson, B. (2004) *Resilient Individuals Use Positive Emotions to Bounce Back from Negative Emotional Experiences.* Journal of Personality and Social Psychology, Vol. 86 No. 2, pp. 320-333

Tyrrell, M., Elliot, R. (n.d.) *The Depression Learning Path.* Available at: www.clinical-depression.co.uk

Vella-Brodrick, D. (2009) *The Relationship Between Goals and Wellbeing.* PowerPoint presentation for IPPA. First World Congress on Positive Psychology. Philadelphia

Wilson, D. (ed.) (2008) *How to Thrive Past 55. What Science tells us about ageing well.* England: Help the Aged.

Wood, S. D. (2012) *United Nations Calls for Happiness-based Economy.* Positive News, Issue 72, Summer

Worthington, Everett L. (2006) *The Path to Forgiveness: Six Practical Sessions for Becoming a More Forgiving Person.* Leader's Manual and Guide. Available at: www.people.vcu.edu/~eworth

Anonymous. *Volunteering boosts self-esteem and wellbeing and helps recovery.* Available at Institute of Psychiatry, Kings College London: www.mentalhealthcare.org.uk

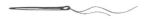

Anonymous. *Why Strengths? The Evidence.* Available at Centre for Applied Positive Psychology: www.CAPPEU.com/portals/3/Files

Excerpt from the poem 'The Invitation' by Oriah from her book, *The Invitation* (c)1999. Published by HarperONE, San Francisco. All rights reserved. Presented with permission of the author. www.oriah.org

Learn a Life Lesson from the Eraser Pencil. Presented with permission of Dr. Everett Worthington www.people.vcu.edu/~eworth

VIA Classification of six virtues and twenty-four character strengths was created by Peterson and Seligman (2004) and is copyright of the VIA Institute on Character. Used with permission. All rights reserved.

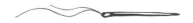

Acknowledgements

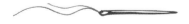

My deepest appreciation, in the first instance, must go to my mother, sister, and daughter – Betty, Pat, and Charlotte – all of whom graciously supported the project and contributed to the Conroy Concept.

Thanks to Oriah Mountain Dreamer, Ryan Niemiec, and Dr. Everett Worthington for allowing me to reproduce their outstanding work. To all the positive psychologists and neuroscientists out there whose ground-breaking research is changing our lives for the better – thank you.

My appreciation to Jack Canfield, Brian Tracy, Deepak Chopra, Dr. Wayne Dyer, Dr. Joe Dispenza, Viktor Frankl, Norman Vincent Peale, and the many others who continue to influence my thinking.

Heartfelt thanks to my brothers and sisters who are always there when needed. A very special thanks must go to Lee (Terrill), my great friend, who reassured and encouraged me almost on a daily basis with her kind words. Where would I be without you?

Last but not least a special thanks to my kids and, of course, to Robin, whose patience and support, especially through the emotional content of the book was, as always, un-ending. Bips.

ABOUT THE AUTHOR

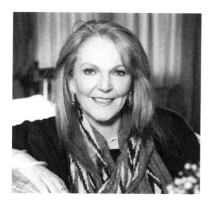

For over twenty-five years Christine Conroy designed furniture to improve the lifestyles of the clients of her family furniture company. Now she transforms her client's lives by designing programmes to help them increase their happiness and well-being. Her interest has always been in helping others to change their lives for better living.

During her forties she transformed her own career by obtaining a First class degree, a Postgraduate Higher Education degree, and going on to become a university lecturer.

It was as a lecturer that Christine realized her students urgently needed personal development guidance. In order to help them, she studied intensively to become a qualified life coach. Since then she has developed a private coaching practice and continues to enjoy leading personal development seminars, lecturing, and public speaking.

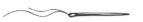

Christine has been married to Robin for thirty-one years and has three grown-up children. She adores her home on the North West Pennine Moors of England and, in addition to helping others find their own happiness, her passions include rich, dark chocolate, and dry stone walls!

If you have questions or comments for Christine on anything you have read in the book; or if you would like her to speak at your event or join one of her courses; she can be contacted through her website at www.ChristineLConroy.com

Remember to download the corresponding workbook to *Stitch Your own Silver Linings* from the website – completely free of charge! (www.ChristineLConroy.com/workbook)

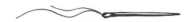

INDEX

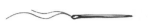